1990

AIDS and the Good Society

Patricia Illingworth

ROUTLEDGE
London and New York

For
Joan Illingworth
Herta Guttman
Margaret Somerville

First published 1990
by Routledge
11 New Fetter Lane, London EC4P 4EE

Simultaneously published in the USA and Canada
by Routledge
a division of Routledge, Chapman and Hall, Inc.
29 West 35th Street, New York, NY 10001

© 1990 Patricia Illingworth

Printed in the Great Britain by
The Guernsey Press Co. Ltd., Guernsey, Channel Islands.

British Library Cataloguing in Publication Data
Illingworth, Patricia
AIDS and the good society. – (Points of conflict).
1. Man. AIDS. Social aspects
I. Title   II. Series
362..1′042

Library of Congress Cataloging in Publication Data
Also available

ISBN 0-415-00023-8 (Hb)
0-415-00024-6 (Pb)

CONTENTS

PREFACE   i

1 THE MORAL CHALLENGE   1

2 RISKY BUSINESS   22

3 SEX, DRUGS AND AUTONOMY   61

4 SOCIAL RESPONSIBILITY   103

5 THE GOOD SOCIETY   137

   WORKS CITED   174

   BIBLIOGRAPHY   180

   INDEX   191

POINTS OF CONFLICT

A new series from Routledge

PREFACE

This book deals with sensitive issues and the conclusions arrived at are ones which many people will find unacceptable. I argue that the prevalence of HIV/AIDS among gay men and IV drug-users can be explained on the basis of social conditions and that in view of this people from these communities who have HIV/AIDS ought to be compensated. My hope is that the arguments which have led to these conclusions will be reflected upon with some care and that, at the very least, they will stimulate further discussion about social responsibility and HIV/AIDS.

In this book, I look at whether or not the behavior that put gay men and IV drug-users at higher risk for HIV/AIDS was performed autonomously and I evaluate AIDS social policy to see if it respects individual autonomy. By analyzing high-risk behavior in terms of whether or not it is performed autonomously I take myself to be partially reflecting values that are endorsed by western societies. At the same time, however, unique emphasis is placed on individual autonomy. Thus, this book constitutes more than just a reflection of currently held values. Rather, I have adopted a liberal framework, which corresponds to at least some of our deeply held convictions about what society ought to be like, and I have considered some of the social problems connected with HIV/AIDS in the light of this framework.

What I have shown in this book is that much of the high-risk behavior of gay men and IV drug-users has not been performed autonomously and that social conditions can account for this high-risk behavior. The view of *autonomy* which I use is instrumental in identifying the social conditions which are, at least, partially responsible for the high concentration of HIV/AIDS in the two communities which I examine. I expect that most people will not agree with the conclusions of this analysis. But, one does not have to endorse liberalism and liberal values to take seriously the claim that social conditions are at the heart of this disease within these two communities. Moreover, as AIDS moves to becoming a classic infectious disease of the poor and disinherited, a deeper understanding of the relationship between AIDS and social conditions is essential. Hence, even readers who strongly disagree with my conclusions about compensation may find something of value in the analysis itself.

Those who endorse other moral frameworks may accept this analysis, but draw different conclusions from it. For example, one might object to the social conditions I identify on purely consequentialist grounds by looking at the harm (AIDS) that these conditions have wrought. This has been done to some extent when I argue that the social conditions which have fostered HIV/AIDS are morally wrong because they harm particular individuals. But, I have also taken this argument a step further by showing that one of the harms caused by the wrongful social conditions is the violation to individual autonomy.

The analysis of high-risk behavior shows that when significant options are reduced people will come to have desires which are inauthentic to them. This, in turn, shows that although people may express a desire for something, the expressed desire does not necessarily reflect their real wishes and may itself be a product of the social context. Thus the analysis of high-risk behavior in terms of whether or not it is autonomous is also important because of the conclusions it leads us to and because of what it reveals about the conditions under which high-risk decisions are made. It shows that although HIV/AIDS is a self-inflicted disease, the *self* involved here is not the autonomous *self*. This has obvious implications for ascriptions of moral responsibility.

I have not shown conclusively that gay men and IV drug-users would not opt for high-risk behavior in the absence of autonomy diminishing social conditions. In the case of gay men some people would argue that multiple anonymous sex, a feature of the sexual lives of many gay men who have HIV/AIDS, is not to be explained by diminished options, but by factors such as freedom from concerns about reproduction. That is, if given an opportunity to make an autonomous choice about how to conduct their sexual lives, free from diminished options, gay men would choose multiple anonymous sex. Some gay men might well make this choice even in ideal circumstances and it may even be the case that many would make such a choice.

It cannot be known with certainty what kind of sexual lifestyle gay men would choose until the social conditions, which stand in the way of a free choice about this matter, disappear. Only then, will it be possible to know how gay men, who currently enjoy the *fast track*, would choose to conduct their sexual lives. The explanation that I give of high-risk behavior is a plausible one and as such it should be taken seriously. The social conditions which I take to foster high-risk behavior are, in any case, unjustifiable from the point of view of liberty and autonomy. Hence, even if the connection between these conditions and HIV/AIDS is disputed, these social conditions ought not to exist.

The focus of this book is on gay men and IV drug-users who have HIV/AIDS. Some people believe that this emphasis only perpetuates the myth that AIDS is a disease of the *other* and consequently the view that it can be ignored by mainstream society. The assumption underlying this objection is that people are only interested in matters which have immediate relevancy to their own case. That is, if a harm such as HIV/AIDS, does not pose a threat to them as individuals, then they will not care about those who are afflicted with it and will not be motivated to improve their situation. It is not at all clear to me that this assumption is true. But if it is a realistic concern, the appropriate response to it is surely not to pander to the lack of compassion on which it is based by underestimating or obscuring the harm to gay men and IV drug-users. Gay men and IV drug-users are focused on here because they have been severely affected by this disease in western societies. This is a sufficient justification to warrant ethical analysis of their situation; to claim that such an analysis is only warranted provided that it is made relevant to other mainstream communities is to fail to value persons for their own sake.

Discussing the moral and social issues which are relevant to gay men and IV drug-users who have HIV/AIDS does not betray a lack of concern for other people who have AIDS any more than discussing feminist issues betrays a lack of concern for the Third World or for Black liberation. I do not mean to discount the compassion which motivates this response with its calls for restrictions on liberty. Compassion for the uniformed adolescent or the helpless neonate is laudable. However, it is misguided to think that restricting autonomy will inevitably lead to maximizing social goodness. It will certainly not lead to an increase in individual autonomy. It is also worth mentioning that I have not adopted gender-neutral language in this book because, at this time and in the West, most of the people with AIDS are men. This practice should not be taken to mean either that women are not at risk for HIV/AIDS or that I am unconcerned about issues having to do with AIDS and women.

The most enjoyable aspect of working in the field of applied ethics is that people, from a wide variety of disciplines and walks of life, are interested in one's research. AIDS research, like research on other pressing social issues, generates interest, discussion and strong opinions. My research has greatly benefitted from the conversations and comments I have had with colleagues friends and loved ones. It is with pleasure that I now turn to the task of thanking them.

This book was written in residence at the McGill Centre for Medicine, Ethics and Law. I am grateful to Margaret Somerville, the Director of the Centre, Richard Cruess, Dean of the Faculty of Medicine, and to my colleagues at the Centre, for the parts that they played in founding the Centre and thus providing a context in which this work could be realized. The Centre provided me with exceptional support, and intellectual and creative stimulation. I am grateful to all of my colleagues at the Centre, but special thanks should go to Norbert Gilmore, Margaret Duckett, Andy Orkin and Ken Morrison for their valuable help. Benjamin Freedman, Michael Hancock and Harold Bursztajn gave me extensive and very insightful comments on earlier drafts of the manuscript as well as a great deal of moral support. I will always be deeply indebted to them.

From the Department of Philosophy, I thank Jim Hankinson and Eldon Soifer, for the care that they took in reading the manuscript and in providing me with comments on it.

Many other people also provided me with useful comments and information. These included Max Allen, Skip Bassford, Alan Bell, David Bloom, Sissela Bok, Lorne Bozinoff, Noah Cowan, Ann Duffie, Sherry Glied, Crystal Green, Lester Grinspoon, Vishwas Govritikar, Mane Hajdin, Julie Hamblin, The Terrence Higgins Trust, Martin Illingworth, Raymond Klibansky, Annette Lefebvre, Merloyd Luddington, Christine Martin, Don Mayo, Richard Mohr, Ethan Nadelmann, Paul Nathanson,

Preface

Ruth Anna Putnam, Peter Singer, Katarina Tomasevski and Morton Weinfeld. To them also I express my gratitude.

I received valuable help from student research assistants. Harold Wilson prepared the index and provided me with substantial comments on the final draft of the manuscript. Victor Ramraj and Rhonda Peterson worked meticulously on the bibliography and notes. I thank each of them for their help.

Those of my readers who expressed profound disagreements with the ideas in this book, but who nonetheless responded to my analysis with time and care, have been personal reminders of the importance of liberal values such as pluralism and tolerance. Special thanks goes to them.

Without the technical skills and patience of Margaret Holding this book would have remained in manuscript form. I am grateful to her for her expert assistance. Gloria Morgan's administrative and organizational talents were also essential for the completion of this book and it is with pleasure that I acknowledge her help and friendship.

I wish also to express my gratitude to Richard Stoneman, from Routledge, Chapman and Hall for encouraging me to write this book and Baruch Brody and the Exxon Educational Foundation for the Exxon Summer Seminar in Medical Ethics. My initial research interest in the fields of Medical Ethics and Philosophy and Social Policy developed out of this seminar.

Much of the research for this book was made possible by a Grant from the National Health Research and Development Program of Health and Welfare Canada. I am grateful to them for their support (number 66052710A2).

1

The Moral Challenge

As of this writing, it has been estimated that world wide over 250,000 people have or have had AIDS (acquired immunodeficiency syndrome) and 5 to 10 million people may be infected with HIV (human immunodeficiency virus), the virus that is known to be linked to AIDS.[1] In the US, as of summer 1988, there have been 66,464 AIDS cases reported to the Centers of Disease Control. A little more than half of these people have died. Since 1981, when reporting began in the US, 63% of people with AIDS have either been homosexual or bisexual men, 7% homosexual or bisexual men with a history of IV drug-use and 19% IV drug-users, both male and female.[2] These figures are staggering. Not in recent memory has a disease wrought so much panic and stimulated so many fantasies. The social and psychological mayhem that has accompanied the discovery of this disease is due largely to circumstances that surround it.

In the West AIDS is most prevalent among highly stigmatized groups: gay men, IV drug-users, Blacks and

1

Hispanics. It is most often fatal and affects people in the prime of their life. The mode of transmission has fostered much of the hysteria associated with AIDS. Homosexuality stirs up deeply embedded fear and aggression.

Discussing how many people have HIV/AIDS and how many have died from it does not strike at the heart of this disease. It makes the pain, suffering and horror of AIDS far too abstract. For the most part, though, this book will be abstract. It will marshall an argument against AIDS social policy which limits the liberty of individuals. The realm of philosophical debate is not meant to appeal to our emotions, nor is it intended to evoke compassion in us.[3] It asks us to examine reasons, and to think logically.

Yet, this disease is having a profound effect on the everyday lives of men, women and children. The suffering and anguish which the human immunodeficiency virus has brought with it, must not be lost sight of. Before turning to the main task of this book it will be helpful to have vividly in mind a picture of the impact of this disease on people.

Life with AIDS

Personal Accounts

One does not actually have to have HIV/AIDS to be profoundly affected by it. Many people, though young gay men stand out here, are terrified that they have AIDS. These people have come to be known as the *worried-well*. Some of them do not know their antibody status and some have been told that it is negative, but do not believe the diagnosis. One man, who asks that his name not be disclosed, described the two years preceding the day that

he was tested and found to be negative for HIV, in much
the same way as someone who actually has the disease
would describe it. For two years this man lived with the
belief that he was HIV positive even though he was not.

> I tried to quit smoking. I tried to quit drinking. I
> became fanatical about exercise and diet. I wanted
> to believe I could beat this numbers game. And I
> cried, to myself and to the very, very few with
> whom I shared the haunting secret.... I was
> unconsciously changing my outlook on everything I
> did, everything I saw. There was no point in
> planning anything long-term - no point in taking on
> new projects at work, no point in developing a
> relationship, no point in dreaming about what I
> wanted to be doing when I was 40, 35 - even 29. I
> couldn't expect to live that long.[4]

This man lived, for all intents and purposes, as if he were
HIV positive. That he did not, in fact, have the disease
made no difference to the anguish he experienced. One
can not help but wonder why he waited for two years to
be tested. His doctor advised him against taking the test
because he was afraid that if his patient were to test
positive 'his name would go on a list and would fall into
the wrong hands'.[5] These fears are not groundless in view
of some of the policies that have either been recommended
or adopted.

If someone endures this much emotional anguish, yet
does not suffer from any of the physical debilities
connected with AIDS, imagine what the situation is for a
person who actually has the disease. Hank Koehn gives
the following account of his experience with AIDS.

> My overpowering fear, now as a man with AIDS,
> was that I would once again be abandoned.... I
> watched my disability grow until I could no longer
> move freely under normal circumstances. I

progressively became more crippled and more useless.... I was being transformed from an independent person into someone who could no longer walk alone, someone who needed help to shower and to get to bed at night.[6]

In his book, *Mortal Embrace*, Emmanuel Dreuilhe illuminates his encounter with AIDS through both military and medical metaphors.

So I wake up every day wondering about the quality of the bowel movements I'll have, which seem magically independent of my diet and the medicines I take. These daily skirmishes are more important and symbolic to me than an overview of the war seen as a whole. And yet the most concrete image of the disease raging in me isn't these bouts of diarrhea revealing the weakening of my intestines. Nor is it the dark spots of Kaposi's .... No, I was first truly seized with terror when I saw a film showing cells magnified millions of times being attacked in vitro by the HIV virus: the speed with which it invaded and captured the cell was chilling, much more so than my own symptoms.[7]

Nor is it only those who have HIV/AIDS or those who consider themselves at high risk for it who are frightened and touched by the disease. The families, friends and lovers of those who have this disease, or feel threatened by it, are also terrified.

The Discovery of AIDS: How One Thing Led to Another

AIDS first came to the attention of the American medical community and, in turn, to the public in 1981.[8] The Centers for Disease Control (CDC) were alerted to the disease by an unusual increase in physician requests for a particular drug, pentamidine, which was then under investigation. Normally, when physicians requested this drug, an account of the conditions warranting the drug and the underlying cause of the condition, accompanied their request. Pentamidine is used to treat people whose immune systems have been severely damaged either by cancer (children receiving chemotherapy for leukaemia often require it) or immunosuppressive drugs.[9] In the case of the recent requests, the condition for which the drugs were being requested was specified, but there was no explanation of why the condition existed. A rare type of pneumonia, *Pneumocystis carinii* pneumonia (PCP), is the condition for which the drug was being requested. Though seeking pentamidine for this particular kind of illness was not unusual, it was not clear why the five young men who needed the drug were suffering from PCP. What was the source of their impaired immune systems? The usual explanations did not work.

At about the same time, the CDC faced a similar challenge with respect to another disease, a rare cancer *Kaposi's sarcoma* (KS). Only a few cases of *KS* had ever been seen in the US, and most of those had been seen in elderly men who had been receiving immunosuppressive treatment. Yet within a thirty-month period, 26 cases had been diagnosed, all among gay men from New York and California, some of whom had also had PCP. Other conditions were also noticed, which were again associated with severely damaged immune systems: chronic lymphadenopathy (enlarged lymph nodes) and a rare kind of lymphoma. Common to all of these relatively rare conditions were age, race, location and sexual orientation.[10] The combination of these features with the panoply of clinical conditions which were characterized by

5

suppressed immune systems made researchers think that there was one underlying cause.[11]

In 1982 this set of conditions came to be known as AIDS. Later in 1983, Luc Montagnier at the Pasteur Institute and Robert Gallo at the National Cancer Institute identified HIV as the infectious agent in AIDS.[12]

In the US, the number of reported AIDS cases was doubling every 6 months. By December 1983 there had been 2,643 cases reported, by April 1985 10,000.[13] The disease is not confined to the US. Many countries in Europe, as well as other parts of the world, have also been affected. As of March 1989, 2,192 AIDS cases have been reported in the UK and 3,494 in Italy. France had a reported 5,655 AIDS cases as of December 1988. As of June 1989, 2,736 people have been reported to have AIDS in Canada and 6,202 in Brazil.[14]

HIV and AIDS

HIV is the name of the virus which is thought to be responsible for AIDS, an end stage disease which is most often fatal. This point needs to be underscored. Not everyone who has HIV has AIDS and it has yet to be shown conclusively that everyone who is HIV positive will get AIDS. It is thought that about 50% of those who are HIV antibody positive will develop full blown AIDS within ten years.[15] In the media, references are often made to the *AIDS virus*, but this is extremely misleading given that it is not known that everyone who is HIV positive will develop it. The virus works by weakening the immune system and, in turn, leaves the body defenceless against the onslaught of opportunistic infections and cancers. At the time of HIV infection a person may experience flu-like symptoms which he may well dismiss as unimportant. Following this, although medical tests could reveal damage to the immune system, the person with HIV might feel perfectly healthy for five or more years.[16] This explains, in part, why HIV/AIDS has spread so rapidly throughout the world. People who carry the virus are often unaware that they carry it and do not feel sick; they do not know that they can infect others. As the virus continues to weaken the immune system patients experience minor opportunistic infections, such as yeast infections of the mouth (thrush) or shingles (*Herpes zoster* infection). As damage to the immune system becomes more severe, major life threatening diseases such as PCP, KS and various kinds of neurological illnesses develop.[17] Loss of weight, diarrhea and intestinal infections are also common with persons who have AIDS.

Transmission

There are three main routes through which a person can come into contact with HIV. First, sexual intercourse, both anal and vaginal, have been shown to transmit the virus, though anal receptive intercourse is thought to be a more efficient mode of transmission than vaginal.[18] Second, a person may become infected through injection (or infusion) of contaminated blood or blood products. In the early history of the disease blood transfusion recipients were at high risk for the virus because they were infused with contaminated blood. By both discouraging those in high-risk groups from donating blood and screening donated blood and plasma for HIV the risk associated with blood products has been dramatically reduced.[19] Now most of those who come into contact with the virus through inoculation are IV drug-users. Infection occurs here by way of contaminated injection equipment (needle-sharing). The third mode of transmission is from infected mothers (usually IV drug-users or the partners of IV drug-users) to their offspring. The fetus comes into contact with the virus while in utero or during birth itself. There is also evidence that the virus can be transmitted through breast milk.

It is important to note about these three routes of transmission that with the exception of injecting the virus into the body (blood transfusion) they are not particularly efficient at transmitting the virus. Researchers Friedland and Klein conclude that:

> The available data indicate that HIV transmission is not highly efficient in a single or a few exposures, unless one receives a very large inoculum. The widespread dissemination of HIV is more likely the result of multiple, repeated exposures over time by routes of transmission that are strongly related to personal and cultural patterns of behavior – particularly, sexual activity and the use of drugs.[20]

The point to be gleaned from this passage is that the chances of contracting HIV/AIDS from a single contact appear to be remote. Social context and lifestyle patterns are the crucial spheres to look at in trying to understand the spread of this virus.

Treatment of Persons with AIDS

At present, there is no cure for HIV/AIDS. Some drug therapies are being used and some are still being investigated and are awaiting approval. Of these, the most promising to date is *azidothymidine* (AZT; now called zidovudine) which has been shown to be effective in prolonging the life of persons with AIDS, decreasing the incidence of opportunistic infections and KS and improving the day-to-day life of persons with the disease.[21] Unfortunately, AZT is often highly toxic. Patients undergoing treatment with it may experience a wide variety of side-effects, including nausea and insomnia; and many people who receive it develop suppression of bone marrow cells or anemia which may require frequent blood transfusions.

Although AZT has improved and prolonged the life of some AIDS patients, it is by no means ideal. The side effects are often difficult for patients to tolerate. The cost is high - about $10,000 (US) per year, per patient. Nor is it known whether AZT is effective at the early stages of infection, although studies have been undertaken on this.[22] A variety of other antiviral drugs are being evaluated for therapy of HIV infection. Interferon and ribavirin are both thought to be promising. Part of the problem faced by both the medical community and persons with AIDS is that the approval of drugs by government is not quick enough to benefit patients who need them. In the US and elsewhere this has given rise to underground networks which provide people who have HIV/AIDS with alternative therapies. The prospect of a vaccine is a long way off and a cure seems remote at this time. Because of these two factors, behavior change is viewed by many people as the only way to cope with the disease now.

HIV/AIDS: A Moral and Social Challenge

HIV/AIDS raises in addition to scientific and medical problems, social and moral ones. Faced with a fatal disease of epidemic proportions social policy-makers must meet the challenge of developing policies which will contain the spread of this virus while at the same time protecting the liberty of individuals. This book is meant as a contribution to that challenge. It by no means lays out answers to all the questions that need to be answered in order to assess various AIDS policy recommendations. In fact the goal of this book is a modest one.

I approach the question concerning what ought to be done about AIDS from within a single philosophical tradition, liberalism. My reasons for using this paradigm of the *good society* are grounded in 1) the sincere belief that liberalism represents more than any other conception of the *good society* an opportunity for people to pursue and enjoy their individual life plans and 2) the belief that most Western societies do more or less try to approximate liberal values.

From the point of view of liberalism, roughly, as articulated by John Stuart Mill, questions about government actions that will interfere with the liberty of individuals must be answered only after a consideration of two matters. First, interference with individual liberty is only justified to prevent the infliction of a harm. But not just any harm will do. The harm must be inflicted on one person by another person. People who harm only themselves with their actions are not to be interfered with. Second, on another version of what constitutes the *good society*, one which is in keeping with the spirit of liberalism, actions which harm only the individual who performs them may also be interfered with if they are not performed autonomously. There are good reasons for this overall restriction on government interference which have to do with what we take human beings to be and the value that we place on them.

Human beings, unlike rocks and lobsters, have the capacity to choose freely. They can be moved to do one thing, reflect on their reasons for wanting to do it, then change their minds and decide to do something else altogether. This capacity for self-reflection distinguishes

10

them from other creatures.[23] Put differently, this capacity gives them the wherewithal to be autonomous, to be self-determining agents.

Because human beings have this unique ability there is an obligation to provide them with as much liberty as possible. Without extensive, wide-ranging and significant options, they cannot be the authors of their own lives.[24] The criterion that is normally invoked to determine how much liberty they ought to have concerns the liberty of others. Each person should be free in so far as his freedom is compatible with the freedom of others. In view of this, the first consideration about when government interference is justified makes perfect sense. By focusing on actions that harm others, it also directs attention to actions which are incompatible with the freedom of others.

In Chapter 2, I look at whether or not the transmission of HIV/AIDS is a case of harm to self or of harm to others.[25] This issue is addressed by looking at both causal and moral responsibility. I conclude that at least within the two highest risk groups, those consisting of gay men and IV drug-users, it is most often a self-inflicted harm. On that ground, and from within a liberal framework, it would be wrong to adopt policies which would interfere with individual liberty. Quarantine, isolation, mandatory and compulsory testing are morally wrong because they interfere with people's claims to do what they want when their actions harm no one but themselves. By showing that people with HIV/AIDS have inflicted this harm on themselves, I thereby show that in the *good society* liberty considerations speak against liberty-limiting social policy.

The claim that we have a moral duty to allow people to harm themselves may strike many people as counter-intuitive. Surely, in the *good society*, we ought to protect people from harm, even that which they inflict on

11

themselves. There are a number of reasons why it is a good idea to resist the temptation to conclude this. First of all, it is not so much that we ought to let people harm themselves as it is that we ought to give them enough freedom to explore different living experiments and life-plans, and sometimes this will entail that they will harm themselves. Two general considerations can be brought forward in support of this: concerns about what is good for individual development and concerns about what is good for the development of society both support this position.[26]

If human beings are viewed as capable of self-authorship and most content when they are able to pursue a life-plan of their own choice and design, it makes sense that we extend to them the freedom needed to cultivate their life-plans. The more options we make available to people, the more likely that they will be able to choose a life-plan which is in concert with how they conceive of themselves. Government interference restricts options and thus restricts the opportunities that people will have to find a way of life which will allow them to express what they regard as essential to themselves.

By allowing people to choose their own life-plans, we not only increase the chance that they will find a life-plan suited to them, but we provide them with crucial opportunities to exercise and hone their uniquely human capacities. John Stuart Mill put this most eloquently in his famous essay "On Liberty".

> He who lets the world, or his portion of it, choose his own plan of life for him has no need of any other faculty than the ape-like one of imitation. He who chooses his plan for himself employs all his faculties. He must use observation to see, reasoning and judgment to foresee, activity to gather materials for decision, discrimination to decide, and when he

has decided, firmness and self-control to hold to his deliberate decision. And these qualities he requires and exercises exactly in proportion as the part of his conduct which he determines according to his own judgment and feelings is a large one.[27]

Mill's point is that if people are not given the liberty to choose how they want to live their own lives they will be denied a crucial opportunity to cultivate essential human faculties. They will be nothing more than automata. A society which, through oppressive legislation and unabiding devotion to what is customary does more than just fail to respect the person (although it certainly does that), it also harms the person. When people are denied opportunities to develop their uniquely human capacities they are harmed.

There are also, of course, benefits to society from a celebration of individual autonomy. It would not be at all surprising if it were the case that people who are self-determining are also creative and original thinkers. If so, then they would contribute more to society than those who are slaves to custom. It may also be that people who are given the opportunity to develop as autonomous individuals tend, in turn, to be more virtuous persons. The combined cultivation of critical faculties and the *moral imagination* may provide the autonomous person with the ability to discern the fine subtleties of moral problems. Those who have not developed these capacities, who take custom as their guide, are less likely to be in a position to identify the moral problems which custom, itself, may generate.

But there is a second consideration which needs to be taken into account and which also has to do with liberty. One objection to taking into account only the question of whether or not an action harms other people is that it ignores the crucial question about whether or not the

13

person who harms only himself does so autonomously. If the reason for not interfering with people's actions is to protect and respect their autonomy, then the actions which they perform and which are protected ought to be autonomous. In Chapter 3, I look at the actions that put gay men and IV drug-users at risk and ask whether or not they are performed autonomously. On the basis of first person accounts, sociological and psychological studies, I conclude that at least in view of one theory of what it is to act autonomously, gay men and IV drug-users, do not, for the most part, autonomously choose in favor of high-risk behavior.

Those who believe that in the *good society* we have an obligation to respect only actions which are performed autonomously might construe this as giving them license to interfere with high-risk behavior. They might argue in the following way. Since the reason for prohibiting interference with actions that harm only the agents of those actions is to protect their autonomy and since on my argument gay men and IV drug-users are not acting autonomously the very considerations that speak against interfering in most cases, speak for it in this case. Namely, a desire to protect individual autonomy. To protect autonomy, bathhouses, gay bars and other venues for high-risk sex ought to be closed. Penalties for narcotic use and trafficking must become stiffer, and the police must become ever more vigilant in their efforts to control drug-use and sodomy.

I argue against this conclusion in Chapter 4 on the grounds that when autonomy is diminished by conditions which mainly have to do with factors outside of the agent's control, such as social conditions, it is the conditions and not the individual which ought to be changed. In the case at hand the obstacles to autonomous decision-making have much more to do with oppressive and repressive social conditions than with conditions which are unique to the individuals who develop HIV/AIDS. Discrimination, poverty, paternalistic and oppressive legislation, all contribute to reducing the options available to gay men and IV drug-users, and in this way, to their high-risk behavior. Were it not for these original infringements on liberty and autonomy, gay men and IV drug-users would not be at higher risk for HIV/AIDS. A negative thesis about what AIDS policy ought to be adopted in the *good society* is advanced. Put differently, I argue that in view of how HIV/AIDS is transmitted and the social circumstances of transmission, it would be wrong to adopt liberty-limiting AIDS social policy.

Another way to look at the argument advanced in this book is as follows. In Chapter 2, I address the first view about when interference is justified and show that with respect to HIV/AIDS interference is not, on that ground, justified. In Chapter 3, I address the second view, that interference is justified when a self-regarding action is not performed autonomously, by looking at whether or not the actions of gay men and IV drug-users are performed autonomously. In Chapter 4, I conclude my analysis of the second view by showing that even according to this strong version of when interference is justified, it is not justified in the case at hand. In this way, I show that according to two socially and philosophically prominent views about when government interference is justified in the *good society*, that it is not justified with respect to the HIV/AIDS epidemic. Together these arguments constitute a strong case against those who would advocate liberty-limiting social policies as a means to stopping the spread of HIV/AIDS in society. My argument shows that the traditional moral justifications for interfering with individual liberty, to protect people from harming either themselves (non-autonomously) or others, are not available in the case of AIDS. To establish them, in spite of this, is to show a complete lack of respect for the autonomy of the individuals concerned. It is to treat them as less than persons.

Out of this negative argument, and the evidence used to buttress it, emerges strong evidence that gay men and IV drug-users have been profoundly harmed. The harms to them are numerous and wide ranging. They have suffered blows to their autonomy and self-esteem; they have endured public ridicule and humiliation by society at large; they have been subjected to discrimination, including loss of jobs, and discriminatory legislation. Gay men have been denied opportunities to cultivate long-term and emotionally satisfying relationships. IV drug-users have, on the one hand, often suffered from socially oppressive and racist conditions which draw them to narcotics and, on the other hand, they are not permitted to pursue this activity unfettered. Both groups have experienced the harm of having their desires manipulated and their claims to autonomy denied.

In Chapter 5, I go beyond a negative thesis and consider what positive duties society has to gay men and IV drug-users who have HIV/AIDS. If I am right, and society has indeed harmed both gay men and IV drug-users, then it has a duty to redress that harm. This, of course, stands over and above the negative duty not to inflict further harm with autonomy diminishing legislation.

I consider the possibility that the forthcoming compensation to persons with HIV/AIDS ought to take the form of enriched and state-funded health care.[28] This proposal is rejected mainly because it is not the most autonomy enhancing form of compensation available to us. I also argue that in countries which already provide for health care it might not serve as compensation at all. Where health care is not provided by the state, it might increase the stigmatization of groups already marked by stigma.

But more importantly, compensation in the form of health care would probably entail that gay men and IV drug-users would have little choice about who cares for them or what kind of care they receive. This point needs to be highlighted. It is important that gay men and IV drug-users have the opportunity to make these decisions not only because they are significant life-decisions and hence autonomy considerations tell in favor of the individual making them, but also because members of these two communities have already suffered enough of a *blow* to their autonomy.

It needs to be kept in mind that those who would be receiving care (gay men and IV drug-users) are the target of widespread discrimination and many of those who would be delivering the care harbor intense prejudices against these people. What is crucial here is not just that gay men and IV drug-users with HIV/AIDS receive the care to which they are entitled, but also that they have some control over who provides that care and how it is delivered.

What is needed is a form of compensation that redresses the harm of HIV/AIDS in a way that allows gay men and IV drug-users to enjoy the dignity associated with the uniquely human capacity to be autonomous. I recommend that they be compensated with money. Unlike other goods, such as health care, money will not tie gay men and IV drug-users to what others want for them - to the conception of the *good* that others take to be worthwhile.

Obligations to gay men and IV drug-users do not rest here. In addition to the duties that I have mentioned, there is also a duty to right any wrongful conditions which have contributed to the harms they have experienced. This, ultimately, is the real moral challenge which the *good society* faces. It will not be easy to replace racism, intolerance and discrimination with tolerance and appreciation of differences. Doing so will require more than just refraining from further harm; positive action will need to be taken.

The most controversial of the conclusions reached in this book hinge on the assumption that considerations of individual autonomy (positive freedom) ought to figure prominently at the macro-level of decision-making. It is only by looking at whether or not high-risk behavior is performed autonomously that we come to understand the role that society has played in the AIDS crisis. In this respect, my approach is to be distinguished from some versions of liberalism, namely, those which rely on a notion of negative freedom. I do, however, show that even on the less polemical criterion of voluntariness, liberty-limiting social policy is not justified in the case of AIDS. Thus, this book speaks to issues which are of concern to both schools of liberalism.

NOTES

1. Jonathan M. Mann, J. Chin, P. Piot and T. Quinn, 'The International Epidemiology of AIDS', *Scientific American*, (October 1988), vol. 259, no. 4, p. 82.

2. William L. Heyward and James W. Curran, 'The Epidemiology of AIDS in the US', *Scientific American*, (October 1988), vol. 259, no. 4, pp. 75, 78.

3. Sometimes we are asked to evaluate arguments, especially moral arguments, by examining our moral intuitions. Although moral intuitions are not decisive with respect to a moral position, they can serve as an initial test of the plausibility of a position.

4. Anonymous, 'A Painful Struggle to Beat The Odds', *Globe and Mail*, Toronto, (December (7) 1987).

5. Ibid.

6. Hank E. Koehn, 'My Passage Through AIDS', *Los Angeles Times*, (August (14) 1987).

7. Emmanuel Dreuilhe, *Mortal Embrace: Living with AIDS*, Linda Coverdale Trans., Hill and Wang, New York, (1988), pp. 103-4.

8. Centers for Disease Control, 'Pneumocystis Pneumonia - Los Angeles', *Morbidity, Mortality Weekly Report*, (1981), vol. 30, pp. 250-2.

9. My discussion of how AIDS was discovered is drawn from two excellent discussions on this topic, see Heyward and Curran, 'The Epidemiology of AIDS in the US', pp. 75-8; and Randy Shilts, *And the Band Played On: Politics, People and the AIDS Epidemic*, St Martin's Press, New York, (1987), pp. 53-69.

10. Heyward and Curran, 'The Epidemiology of AIDS in the US', p. 74.

11. Ibid., p. 74.

12. Ibid., p. 75.

13. John Green and David Miller, *AIDS: The Story of a Disease*, Grafton Books, London, (1986), pp. 20-1.

14. Federal Centre for AIDS, 'Surveillance Update: AIDS in Canada', Federal Centre for AIDS, Health and Welfare Canada, Ottawa, (June (5) 1989).

15. George Rutherford, 'HIV Infection: Outcome and Survival', *Proceedings of International Symposium on the Economic Impact of HIV Infection in Canada*, (forthcoming publication of the McGill Centre for Medicine, Ethics and Law).

16. Norbert Gilmore, 'Patient Care for AIDS', *Transplantation/ Implantation Today*, (September 1988), vol. 5, p. 47.

17. Ibid.

18. It is also thought that men transmit the virus much more effectively to women than women to men. It has been suggested that this point may be important in understanding why some people maintain that HIV/AIDS is not a problem for heterosexuals. It may be that once again *sexism* rears its ugly head. If male to female transmission is more effective than female to male, then heterosexual women may be at greater risk for HIV/AIDS than would heterosexual men. Thus the perception that HIV/AIDS is not a problem for heterosexuals may be colored by the fact that it is less of a problem for heterosexual men than heterosexual women. I wish to thank Margaret Somerville for bringing this point to my attention.

19. Gerald H. Friedland and Robert S. Klein, 'Transmission of the Human Immunodeficiency Virus', *New England Journal of Medicine*, (October (29) 1987), vol. 317, no. 18, p. 1125.

20. Ibid., p. 1133.

21. Norbert Gilmore, 'Patient Care for AIDS', p. 48.

22. Ibid.

23. See Harry Frankfurt, 'Freedom of Will and Concept of a Person', *Journal of Philosophy*, (1971), vol. 68, pp. 5-20.

24. For an excellent discussion of the importance of a wide range of significant options for autonomy, see Joseph Raz, *The Morality of Freedom*, Clarendon Press, Oxford, (1986), pp. 369-95.

25. This question was first addressed by Richard D. Mohr in 'AIDS, Gays and State Coercion', *Bioethics*, (1987), vol. 1, no. 1, pp. 35-50. Unlike Mohr I raise this question about *both* gay men and IV drug-users. Although I agree with the conclusion Mohr arrives at, I provide different arguments in support of it.

26. See John Stuart Mill, 'On Liberty', in *John Stuart Mill: On Liberty*, E. Rapaport, ed., (Introduction by E. Rapaport), Hackett Publishing Co., Indianapolis, (1978).

27. John Stuart Mill, 'On Liberty', p. 56.

28. Richard Mohr argued for this view, with respect to gay men, in *Gays/Justice: A Study of Ethics, Society and Law*, Columbia University Press, New York, (forthcoming).

2
Risky Business

Sex, Drugs and Decisions

In Germany, the Bavarian government has a policy of mandatory blood testing for prostitutes, drug addicts, prisoners, public sector job applicants and foreigners seeking residence and work permits. Belgium requires third world scholarship students to be tested; those who test positive lose their scholarship and are sent home. The leader of France's right-wing National Front party has called for twice yearly screening of all French citizens with mandatory follow up for those who test positive. The proposal also recommends confinement in *special AIDS clinics* for confirmed AIDS cases. In Costa Rica hospitals provide health authorities with the names of patients they believe should be tested for antibodies. In Sweden, pharmacists distribute free sterile needles to IV drug-users and a *lovebus* tours beaches and vacation spots dispersing, among other things, AIDS awareness literature and free condoms. The Swedish government mailed condoms to

240,000 men and women between the ages of 18 and 24. Needles without prescription can be had by IV drug-users in Britain, France, Italy and the Netherlands among other nations.[1]

This is just a sample of how different countries are trying to cope with HIV/AIDS. These measures, debated or put into effect, are in some cases highly intrusive of individual liberty, while other measures are liberty enhancing. Measures of this sort, designed primarily to stop the spread of HIV/AIDS, need to be evaluated on the basis of two criteria: whether or not they can be morally justified and how effectively they control the spread of the disease. That moral considerations must come into play is obvious. The most effective way to stop the spread of HIV/AIDS might be to round up all those who test positive and who have AIDS, and then give them a painless but lethal injection. Although highly effective, few would defend such a measure and in support of their refusal to do so they would cite moral considerations. This point needs to be underscored. Measures for checking the spread of this disease need to be assessed on the basis of both moral considerations and effectiveness.

For these ends to be accomplished, the actions that are high risk for AIDS must be understood. It is important to know not just what actions put people at risk for HIV/AIDS, but also why people perform them. That is, the motives and reasons underlying high-risk behavior need to be studied. This information will be helpful for a moral evaluation of policies because it will allow us to assess whether or not the high-risk actions of those in high-risk groups are autonomous. If so, and if they are also self-regarding actions, then given the value placed on autonomy in the *good society*, it is wrong to interfere with them. From the point of view of the effectiveness of proposed AIDS measures, it is useful to know the reasons behind high-risk activities because this information can be instrumental in determining appropriate ways for decreasing high-risk behavior. For example, if the only reason IV drug-users share equipment is because they do not have easy access to new equipment, it would certainly be effective to provide them with free sterilized equipment.[2]

In the two highest risk groups, gay men and IV drug-users, individuals perform actions which place them at higher risk for HIV/AIDS: either they have unprotected (anal) sex or they share injecting equipment with others. Were they to abstain from performing these actions they would dramatically reduce their chances of developing HIV/AIDS. In the case of HIV/AIDS the actions of individuals are crucial.

The Harm Principle

Two important questions need to be addressed before the moral worthiness of particular AIDS policies can be assessed: 1) Is HIV/AIDS transmitted within the two high-risk groups primarily through actions which are self-regarding or other-regarding? Another way to understand this, is in terms of harm to self (self-regarding actions) and harm to others (other-regarding actions). 2) If the actions by which the virus is transmitted are self-regarding, and cause no harm other than that to which the individual consents, has the individual acted autonomously?

The first question is important because, in the *good society*, there is a general reluctance to interfere with people's liberty unless it is absolutely necessary. One way to restrict the number of occasions for interfering is to interfere only when an action harms others. This is known as the *harm principle* (I refer to it as the *strong harm principle*). If an action causes harm only to the individual who performs it, then on the basis of the *strong harm principle* interference is unjustified. I will argue in this chapter that HIV/AIDS is transmitted primarily through self-regarding actions.

The second question, which will be addressed in Chapter 3, is important because according to another principle, the *weak harm principle*, even when someone inflicts harm only on himself, it is important that he does so autonomously.[3] If a self-inflicted harm is not autonomously chosen, then interference may be warranted just so that the conditions which stand in the way of an autonomous choice are removed. Sometimes, this will require providing a person with information. At other times, the conditions, either social or psychological, which are obstacles to autonomy, may have to be removed.

Thus, according to the *strong harm principle*, the rightness or wrongness of interfering with an action depends on whether or not that action harms other people. When an action does harm others without their consent, the state may interfere with it; steps may be taken to prevent the person from performing it. According to John Stuart Mill, this is a necessary condition for interfering. He also believed that it needs to be shown that the proposed interference will be efficacious.[4] This caveat has important implications for social policy. For a liberty-limiting policy to be put into practice it must not only achieve the end for which it is designed, but the proposed interference must not cause more harm than it prevents. The efficacy caveat must be met even when the action for which interference is proposed is an other-regarding one (harms other people). A number of people concerned with AIDS social policy have shown that liberty-limiting AIDS policies, such as isolation, mandatory testing and reporting are inefficient and might well cause more harm than good.[5]

Persons with HIV/AIDS experience harm. Knowing only this, however, is not very helpful in determining what AIDS social policy ought to be adopted if, at the same time, either version of the *harm principle* is to be respected. In addition to knowing that there is a harm, it is important to know how that harm has come about. In this chapter, I consider how individuals with HIV/AIDS have been harmed, but also how, if at all, society has been harmed by the AIDS epidemic. Thus AIDS raises the possibility of harms to both particular individuals and to the collective, in this case, a harm to the public health.

Harm to Particular Individuals

Harm
People experience harms either through their own actions or the actions of others. Is the transmission of HIV/AIDS from one person to another a case of one person harming another or a case of one person harming him or herself?[6] The following simplified examples will illuminate this basic distinction.

Harm to Others
Jack takes out a gun, pulls the trigger and shoots Sue. Sue dies as a consequence of his action. There is no room for doubt about the source of the harm to Sue. Jack harms her. His action is other-regarding; it has a direct and harmful consequence for Sue. In view of the harm to Sue, Jack's action is clearly an other-regarding one.

Harm to Self

Alternatively, suppose that Jack takes out a gun, pulls the trigger and shoots not Sue, but himself. Jack dies. Imagine also that Jack has no dependents and no friends. Here his action qualifies as a self-regarding one. He harms only himself.

Consent to Harm

Imagine a third variation on this example. This time Sue tells Jack that she is dying of cancer and pleads with him to shoot her. Jack does and she dies. In this case Sue consents to the harm that befalls her. So although she is harmed, she is, in a morally relevant way, the agent of the action that harms her. This would seem to be a case of self-harm. It is important to notice here that even though Jack is the instrument of harm, Sue is the agent of it.

The high-risk actions of gay men and IV drug-users fit most comfortably into this third category. Although gay men and IV drug-users do not consent explicitly to harm in the way that Sue does, they do perform actions which imply *consent*. This third category of actions, though perhaps counter-intuitively, qualify as harm to self. A legal maxim, *volenti non fit injuria* will help to explain why, though paradoxically, this is so. Translated as "To one who consents no harm is done" the *volenti* maxim is obviously false in one sense; an individual can certainly be harmed by an action to which he consents. Joel Feinberg suggests that we understand the *volenti* maxim as not concerned with *harms* but with *wrongs* and injustices. On this interpretation the maxim means something like the following: To one who freely consents to a thing no *wrong* is done, no matter how harmful the consequences may be.[7] The point here is that someone who has consented to harm cannot afterward complain that he has been wronged. Another, though paradoxical way to look at the matter, is

27

that someone who consents to x, does not regard x as a harm even though others do. One man's harm is another man's pleasure.

IV Drug-Users, AIDS and Self-Inflicted Harm

IV drug-users are the second largest high-risk group in the US and in other developed countries where HIV/AIDS is a problem (Britain for example). It is primarily through IV drug-users that HIV/AIDS extends to non-high-risk groups. Approximately three-quarters of the heterosexuals with AIDS have had sexual relations with an IV-user.[8] The incidence of reported AIDS cases is increasing among IV drug-users; it appears to be stabilizing in the gay community.[9] Stopping the spread of the disease in the drug community poses a serious problem for policy makers. The activity that puts IV-users at risk is sharing injection equipment (*works*). For reasons which I will look at more closely in the next chapter, needle-sharing is a common practice among IV-users. Through injection equipment the virus is passed from one IV-user to another; then perhaps from an IV-user to a sexual partner and in the case of women, possibly on to their offspring.

For an IV-user to become infected with HIV/AIDS, the injection equipment he uses must be contaminated with the virus. If an infected IV-user shares his equipment with others, then there is a very good chance that they too will become infected with HIV (provided that they don't sterilize the equipment). There is nothing mysterious about how the virus is transmitted among IV-users. Less perspicuous, is whether or not transmission of the virus from the infected user to others, and the harm to them, qualifies as an instance of a self-inflicted harm or a harm inflicted on one by another. I shall argue that with respect to both *causal* and *moral responsibility* the mode of transmission of HIV is firmly situated in the domain of self-harm among IV-users.

Causal Responsibility

Consider a hypothetical example between Smith and Jones. Smith who is HIV positive has a set of *works* which he shares with Jones. Jones after using Smith's equipment becomes HIV positive. Smith is instrumental in contaminating the needle that Jones later inserts into his vein. Does this show that Smith is causally responsible for the harm to Jones?

Certainly, Smith's action of using and contaminating the equipment cannot be what harms Jones. After all, Jones subsequently took the equipment from Smith and used it himself. It is important to bear in mind that Jones is only harmed after he takes the needle and inserts it into one of his veins. For Smith to be causally responsible for what happens to Jones, he would have to be causally responsible for the fact that Jones uses his equipment. Surely, he is not. Special circumstances aside, Jones's action of inserting the needle into his vein would seem to count as his own action and the harm that results from it a self-inflicted one.

Unlike the above case of self-inflicted harm, a harm by one to another, would go as follows: had Smith thrown Jones to the ground, grabbed him by the arm and thrust the contaminated needle into his throbbing artery (contrary to Jones's desires), Smith would certainly have caused the harm. Jones does nothing to cooperate with Smith in the activity. He is a victim of Smith's wickedness. In the earlier case, however, Jones is the agent of the action which harms him.

29

Normally, an individual's agency in a causal chain is taken to break that chain and to initiate a new act.[10] Some people (although by no means all) would qualify this by saying that when there is a clear intention to involve the actions of another in the harm, this principle no longer applies. Whether or not one endorses this caveat is not all that important in the case of IV drug-users because there is little reason to think that they would, for the most part, use HIV infection as a mechanism for harm.

Moral Responsibility

Even if Smith sets out to harm Jones, it is not clear that he is morally responsible for the harm to Jones. The moral intuition underlying the *volenti* maxim is that if an individual consents to a harm, he is not wronged. Although Jones certainly doesn't consent to HIV infection in the way that Sue consents to be shot by Jack, it is plausible that he does consent to the risk of it. This would be so if, at the time that he decides to engage in high-risk sex, he can foresee the risk of HIV infection. Foreseeability would rest on when in the history of the AIDS epidemic the Jones/Smith encounter took place and how much information was available about HIV.

This line of reasoning might give rise to the following objection.[11] Surely, if Jones does not know Smith's antibody status he cannot consent to the harm which follows his action. When an IV drug-user consents to the risk of coming into contact with HIV through contaminated equipment he consents only to a specific risk, to be determined by the prevalence of the virus among IV drug-users in general. If, for example, 10% of addicts are HIV positive he consents to only a 1 in 10 chance of coming into contact with this virus in each encounter of needle-sharing. If it turns out that the first contact is HIV positive, then the drug-user may allege not to have consented to the risk of HIV because he has only consented to a 10% chance of coming into contact with it. To support this position he might urge that he can only consent to what he knows and as far as he knows his chances of getting HIV are 1 in 10.

This is an interesting, though naive objection. It cannot be the case that when someone consents to a 10% risk, he holds the false belief that when he shares equipment he risks contracting HIV exactly 1 out of 10 times, that is, that he has 9 free times. Surely he must realize that risks are not evenly distributed across a specific population. If Jones shares a needle with 10 other people he must do so knowing that perhaps everyone or no one is HIV positive. It would, frankly, be foolish to think otherwise.[12]

The question of whether or not Smith is morally responsible for the harm to Jones does not rest with the issue of consent. For Smith to have wronged Jones he would also have to have a moral duty to Jones to inform him that the injection equipment might be contaminated. There is a good argument to support the view that no such duty exists.[13]

I will argue, using a consequentialist framework, that with respect to gay men and IV drug-users, in high-risk circumstances, there is no duty to disclose HIV status. Contextual considerations are important for a consequentialist analysis of moral duties because they are crucial for determining whether a proposed duty will produce more harm than good. Moral duties which are, for instance, unlikely to be satisfied, can be counter-productive. People may be left confused, frustrated and disappointed. The potential harm from duties which generate expectations, but which remain unfulfilled, needs to be taken into account in the case of the duty to disclose

HIV status to see whether or not gay men and IV drug-users, who participate in high-risk activities, have a duty to each other to disclose their HIV status.

There is not sufficient trust within the high-risk relationships of gay men and IV drug-users to ground a duty to disclose. I will show that neither gay men nor IV drug-users who participate in high-risk activities expect co-participants to disclose their HIV status. On this line of reasoning, from the fact that there is no expectation that others will disclose their HIV status, it follows that there is no trust with respect to disclosure and, in turn, that there is no duty to disclose HIV status.

I assume that the absence of an expectation to disclose HIV status is evidence that there is a lack of trust in others that they will disclose their status. Consider the following example. Most of us expect other people, even passing strangers, to tell us the time of day when we ask them. This expectation is one that is easily satisfied and does not require any sacrifice or inconvenience on the part of other people; trust comes easily in this case. That we do trust people to give us the correct time is evidenced by the fact that we do not normally try to confirm the truth of their response.

The same is not true for other sorts of expectations, especially expectations which require some sacrifice on the part of other people for their satisfaction and which entail a high cost to those who hold these expectations when they are not satisfied. For instance, not many people would disclose highly personal information to a complete stranger. The absence of an expectation that others will keep one's secrets bears witness to the lack of trust in others with respect to very private matters. Gossips, for example, cannot be trusted with deep dark secrets and so we do not form expectations that they will be able to maintain confidentiality. On the other hand, close friends are expected to be trustworthy when it comes to personal information and we do expect them to keep our confidence. Friends, unlike strangers, have earned our trust by meeting our expectations. There is a reciprocal relationship between trust and expectations such that as our expectations are met by others our trust in them grows. Similarly, as our trust grows, our expectations rise. Hence, the amount of trust that exists between them can serve as an indication of what expectations they will have of one another and the expectations they have can serve as an indication of the trust that exists between them.[14]

In general, people do not come to have expectations which are unlikely to be satisfied and the amount of trust that exists between them is one of the considerations that they take into account before formulating their expectations. This would seem to be just a matter of prudence. If people are not trustworthy, then expectations are likely to go unfulfilled and unfulfilled expectations have undesirable consequences. When the failure to satisfy an expectation has serious consequences, as it would in the case of expectations to disclose HIV status, the level of trust required for the formulation of an expectation will be greater than it would be otherwise[15].

This analysis will help to shed light on the Smith and Jones example. Smith would be morally responsible for the harm to Jones if he has a moral duty to inform Jones that the equipment is contaminated and does not fulfil it. If Smith does have such a duty to Jones, the harm to Jones would no longer qualify as a harm to self.[16] If, for instance, an alcoholic has a family and his alcoholism interferes with his ability to meet his moral obligations to them, his drinking is other-regarding. It is other-regarding because he has an assignable duty of care for them. Is it the case that individuals, who might next use the contaminated equipment, have some kind of moral claim on others to inform them about their antibody status? Is there, among IV drug-users, an expectation that others will disclose their HIV status? The question of whether or not an IV-user has a moral duty to inform another IV-user of his antibody status turns on the answer to this empirical question.

In a friendship, mutual trust of some minimal amount is taken for granted; there is an assumption that friends do not wilfully attempt to harm one another and that they will try to enhance each others' good.

Does mutual trust characterize the friendships that exist in the drug community? I think not. The following passage taken from an autobiographical essay written by Dennis Waltington, an ex-drug-addict, is instructive on this point.

> "Dennis! Hey, man, what's up with you?" I turn and see, seated on the landing above, my old friend Michael ...
> My first instinct is to avoid him, as I do everyone from my past, but I see immediately from Michael's dramatic weight loss that he has also been hooked by the Master (Crack). The drug has deflated his massive frame.
> "Hey, man, you slidin' down the same pole I'm on," Michael says.
> "I guess I am," I say. "You know where I can cop?"...
> "You have full money?"
> "Yeah. Sixty-five dollars."
> "Damn, nigger, you must not have been out here too long," says Michael.
> "What you mean?" I ask.
> "Calling out what you got in your pocket," he replies. Then he grins and hugs me in a brotherly fashion....
> We enter the building and climb a flight of stairs. Suddenly, Michael darts ahead of me as I feel the

weight of two men behind me forcing me against the wall. One instructs, "Don't breath." The other pulls a gun, places it to my temple, pressing my head against the wall. At the same time, Michael places a knife to my throat and jabs it lightly on the vein. They take my money, cigarettes, and shoes. Michael says, "I'm sorry, man, but you can't trust old friends who's into the Rock."[17]

There is a moral to be drawn from this story. Although Waltington trusted his friend, Michael, he was wrong to do so. Friendship, as a relationship of mutual trust, is difficult to achieve when at every turn one's expectations are disappointed. Waltington is unlikely to extend his trust quite so rapidly in the future and though he may continue to count Michael as among his friends, he will, as Michael, himself cautions, not trust him.

Paradoxically *friendship* and *mistrust* appear to be compatible in the relationships that drug-addicts form. These *friendships* obviously do not generate and nurture trust. They are ambivalent: on the one hand there are warm and benevolent emotions and, on the other hand, a willingness to exploit those same sentiments for quick gain.[18] Let's face it, the life of a drug-addict is not a life for the faint of heart. It is a world which contains the euphoric pleasures of narcotics, but also one which contains a number of risks, the risk of social isolation, the risk of legal repercussion, risks associated with the narcotic itself - and, of course, the risks associated with dealing with people associated with narcotics. IV drug-users can expect to encounter people from the underworld, undercover narcotics agents and informers. Their world, fraught with treachery, is not conducive to mutual trust and concern.

A certain minimum of interpersonal trust is needed to conduct the business of providing drugs and the equipment and locations for injecting, and for the social validation of the worth of *getting high*. The interpersonal trust is in precarious balance with a generalized mistrust among members of the IV-drug use subculture. Among the many reasons for this mistrust are competition for scarce goods (drugs and the money to buy them), use of informants by law enforcement agencies, carryover of the *hustling* of *straights* to the hustling of other drug-users, and the use of violence to settle disputes.[19]

There are far too many uncertainties and ambiguities in the drug community for IV drug-users to form an expectation that other IV-users will disclose their HIV status. For this reason, there is no duty to disclose. In view of this, moral considerations do not tell in favor of moral responsibility for HIV transmission among IV drug-users.[20]

With respect to individual IV-users, HIV is transmitted primarily through individual actions and responsibility for the harm, HIV/AIDS, falls on the shoulders of the individual who performs it and not on others. If this is so, then, transmission of HIV/AIDS in the drug sub-culture falls, for the most part, into the category of self-harm and not into that of harm to others.[21]

Gay Men, AIDS and Self-Inflicted Harm

A similar line of reasoning applies to HIV transmission in the largest high-risk group, the gay male community. In a paper entitled "AIDS, Gays, and State Coercion", Richard Mohr defends the thesis that AIDS is transmitted through a voluntary act and that this act harms no one other than those who consent to it.[22] He believes that transmission of the virus among gay men is primarily a case of harm to self. On the basis of this, he concludes that government would be wrong to regulate behavior which is basically private. Assessing whether or not an act is performed voluntarily does not exhaust the issue of ascribing responsibility for it, especially when the conditions for what constitutes a *voluntary* act are not specified. Mohr's early application of, what is in effect, the *harm principle*, while enlightening, is nonetheless incomplete with respect to questions of autonomy. As I show in the next chapter an action can be voluntary yet not autonomous. At this time, however, I want only to strengthen Mohr's view that transmission of HIV among gay men is a case of self-harm.

Causal Responsibility

Gay men come into contact with HIV primarily through sexual activity. Anal receptive intercourse with multiple anonymous partners is thought to be particularly risky.[23] Consider, first, a straightforward *harm to others* case, in which one man's action has harmful consequences for another. Homosexual rape, a frequent occurrence in many prisons, is often aggressive and violent.[24] Imagine that someone who is HIV positive rapes another man and transmits the virus to him.[25] Here sex is not cooperative; it is against the will of the person who is raped. The rape victim is harmed in so far as his claims to privacy and self-determination are violated and he may now be infected with HIV.[26]

Rape is a clear-cut case of one person causing a harm to another.[27] The action of one man directly harms another man; his action is an other-regarding one. If the virus is transmitted through rape, the victim has been harmed by another. Although there are certainly instances within the gay community in which the virus is transmitted through violent means, these instances would account for only a small fraction of HIV/AIDS cases within the gay community.

Now consider a less clear-cut example. Imagine that it is the summer of 1987 and Sam, a gay man, goes to a local park in Los Angeles which is well known for gay cruising. There he has sex with four other men. One of these men, Bob, is someone who cruises frequently and who eschews safe sex practices. The same is true for Sam. Unbeknownst to Sam, Bob is HIV positive and during this particular tryst the virus is transmitted to Sam. Would it be accurate to say that in transmitting the virus to Sam, Bob harms him, that Bob is causally responsible for the harm to Sam? This case is different from the rape case because here the person to whom the virus is transmitted is a willing partner, and in the other, he is not. Sex between Bob and Sam is cooperative, just as the sharing of injection equipment is between Jones and Smith. Think of the *volenti* maxim again. Someone who consents to a harm is not wronged.

But does Sam consent to be harmed? In one sense, he does. After all, Sam went to the park looking for impersonal sex. If he was seeking such an encounter and through gestures or whatever indicated to Bob that he was interested in impersonal sex then Sam consented, if he did not initiate the encounter with Bob. Because of this, and in virtue of the *volenti* maxim, it would seem that he is not wronged by Bob.

Sam shows a desire and willingness to have sex with Bob. To see if he consents to the harm, it needs to be decided if the possibility of infection was a foreseeable consequence of his action. The example, as I describe it, is designed to include information which is relevant to the reasonable person criterion of foreseeability.[28] For instance, I specify that Sam is cruising in a major US city in the summer of 1987. In view of this, it is difficult to imagine that he is unaware, or should not have been aware, that he is risking contact with HIV/AIDS. Surely, any reasonable person in Sam's position would know that HIV infection is a possible consequence of the action he performs with Bob. In other words, it is reasonable to assume that Sam foresees that HIV infection might be a consequence of his action. Given this, it would seem to follow that Sam consents not only to have sex with Bob, but to have high-risk sex with him. If so, then Sam's harm is a self-inflicted one.[29]

To undermine this argument, one might argue that it is unreasonable to think that anyone would consent to risk HIV infection and the possible consequence of it, AIDS. Hence, there is *prima facie* evidence that Sam would *not* consent to high-risk sex and, therefore, could not have foreseen the possible harm connected with his action. If Sam had foreseen the consequence of his action he would not have consented to it. This argument ignores the panoply of sexual desires and tastes that people actually have. There is no reason to think that some people do not desire risky sex and the excitement that goes along with it.[30] To assert otherwise is just to be arbitrary and blind to the diversity of sexual desire. People are just not as rational in formulating their desires as this argument would have them.

Although some gay men may have a desire for risky sex, many of those who eschew safer sex practices may do so because they have an interest which competes with their interest in safer sex.[31] For instance, some gay men may find that taking time to slip a condom on interrupts passion or that condoms diminish feelings of pleasure.[32] Even if this is so, and it is not risk *per se* which is sought, these men would seem to consent to risk in order to obtain something which they value more (passion and/or pleasure). People willingly incur risks of this sort all the time. Smokers, for example, risk their health for the pleasure of nicotine.

Moral Responsibility

Suppose that, contrary to what I have argued, Bob is causally responsible for the harm to Sam. This would be so, for instance, if a reasonable person would not foresee that HIV infection is a possible consequence of a sexual encounter of the sort I described. That someone is causally responsible for inflicting a harm on another person is not, though, in and of itself, enough to take the harm out of the *harm to self* category. It also needs to be asked whether or not the person is morally responsible for the harm.

With respect to IV drug-users, I argued that in the absence of a widespread expectation to disclose HIV status, there is no duty to disclose. The same considerations are relevant for identifying whether or not gay men have a duty to disclose their HIV status to one another. I will argue that it is unlikely that impersonal sexual encounters among gay men generate an expectation that partners will disclose their HIV status.

It is an empirical question whether or not gay men entering into impersonal sexual relations expect their partners to inform them of the possible harms the encounter might hold for them.[33] By looking at the nature of impersonal sexual relationships, we can see what expectations they are likely to create. Gay men seeking impersonal sex are, for the most part, trying to minimize personal contact. Anonymity is often an important part of the pleasure of the encounter. In many of these encounters there is no exchange of words; sometimes only gestures are used as a means of indicating a desire for sex or to show pleasure and gratitude. Yet, information about a partner's antibody status is of a highly personal and confidential nature. Revealing it might open doors which are not in keeping with the overall intent of the encounter; it might make the encounter, as conceived, impossible. Thus, disclosure of one's antibody status may be incompatible with impersonal sex.

Consider the case of Sam and Bob again. On the one hand, Sam might assume that Bob is basically beneficent toward his partners and that if there were a possibility of harm, he would be forthright and inform Sam of it. Surely it is unreasonable for Sam to think that Bob, a complete stranger, is beneficent, especially given the confusion Bob may have about what Sam desires. For instance, Bob might assume that if Sam were particularly concerned about HIV infection, he would not be cruising in parks prepared to have unsafe sex. If what Sam wants is high-risk sex, then he may not want this information. Bob might also think that if what Sam wants is highly impersonal sex, then he may not want to engage in the kind of discussion that would be required to convey information about antibody status. In any case, it is unlikely that Sam would expect a stranger to be direct and honest with him about a matter so very personal.

This claim is supported by practices within the gay community. Gay men have encouraged and stood strongly behind safe sex as the appropriate response to the AIDS crisis. In San Francisco, for example, during the mid-eighties, it was customary for gay men to wear safety pins on their lapels to signal to other men that they practice safe sex. It is interesting, from the point of view of this discussion, that they signaled their endorsement of safe sex and not their antibody status. It would be reasonable to suppose that gay men recognize that it is much more likely that people will be truthful about their sexual conduct than about their HIV status. This shows that, within the gay community, there is not a widespread expectation that people will disclose their antibody status. In fact, one could interpret the emphasis placed on safe sex as positive evidence that gay men expect that others will not tell them that they are HIV positive. It may be that some gay men *hope* that their sexual partners will inform them of their antibody status and it might be *nice* of them to do so. But in the absence of a widespread expectation to disclose, neither of these will suffice to ground a *duty* to disclose HIV status.

The crux of the matter is that a duty to disclose HIV status would not be in the interest of gay men because it might do more harm than good by creating expectations that will not be satisfied and by taking the responsibility for infection of HIV/AIDS out of the hands of individuals who are, in fact, vulnerable to it. To posit a duty to inform implies that the responsibility for transmission lies with the infected rather than with the uninfected to remain uninfected. This, in turn, may have the consequence of making the uninfected take fewer precautions to avoid HIV infection. For instance, if Sam believes that it is Bob's moral responsibility to inform him of his antibody status, he may construe Bob's silence as an invitation to not practice safe sex. He may be working on the assumption that if safe sex were necessary, Bob would inform him.

Positing a duty to inform about one's antibody status may well lead to a reduction in the practice of safe sex in the gay community and thus to a rise in the spread of HIV/AIDS. The gay community has adopted safe sex as a solution to the spread of HIV/AIDS and not moral duties to inform.[34] From a consequentialist point of view, it would be counter-productive to posit such a duty.

There is another reason why it is unreasonable to think that impersonal sexual encounters generate a duty to disclose. A duty to inform relevant others about one's antibody status would entail that a gay man know his antibody status.[35] Many people may not want this information and for good reason. Knowledge about one's antibody status may cause severe depression and anxiety and it may not lead to a reduction in high-risk behavior.[36]

Consider the following. A gay man may know of himself that he is more effectively motivated to comply with safer sex guidelines through self-interest than altruism and that, given this, he would rather not know his antibody status. Put differently, he might believe that he should practice safe sex and he might know that the most effective form of motivation for him is the self-interested desire to protect himself from coming into contact with HIV/AIDS. But he also knows of himself that if he knows that he tests positive he will be discouraged from practicing safe sex. So he decides to remain ignorant of his antibody status.

This scenario suggests that some gay men may have very good reasons for not wanting information about their antibody status. The point is that it is far from clear that knowing one's antibody status will decrease one's high-risk activity. The decision about whether or not it will is one for the individual gay man to make because he is probably in the best position to know what sort of considerations most effectively motivate him. If this is true, then there is further reason to believe that it would not be in the best interest of the gay community to posit a duty to inform.

In response to this line of reasoning, it might be argued that the duty to inform does not apply to everyone, but only to those who know that they are HIV positive. If this were so, then people who are most effectively motivated to practice safe sex by ignorance of their HIV status would not be placed in the counter-productive position of having to know their antibody status. The problem with this proposal is that it would provide some gay men with grounds for not taking the test for HIV. Some gay men may 1) need to know that they are HIV positive to practice safe sex, and 2) may not want to disclose a positive test result to others. If these people are morally obligated to disclose the results of a positive test, then they may well decide to avoid the test altogether. By providing them with a reason to remain ignorant of their antibody status, we may also be denying them the very mechanism they need to practice safe sex, namely, knowledge that they are HIV positive. Hence, even this modified version of the duty to inform may turn out to be counter-productive.

Let me rehearse the discussion of the last few pages. I showed that the transmission of HIV among gay men, who participate in the *fast track*, falls, for the most part, into the category of self-harm. I argued that gay men do not expect to be informed of a partner's antibody status and hence that there is not a moral duty to disclose such information. I showed that impersonal sexual encounters are not conducive to an expectation that others will disclose. I also suggested that it would be counter-productive to posit a duty to disclose HIV status.

Individuals who practice unsafe impersonal sex take their fate into their own hands. At a certain stage in the history of HIV/AIDS, most gay men knew their status as members of a high-risk group for AIDS, and they knew what measures they had to take to avoid the disease. This is important because it shows that the practice of unsafe sex, at one stage in the genesis of AIDS, is a self-inflicted harm and ought not to be interfered with on that ground. The idea that there is an assignable duty to inform partners of one's antibody status is problematic for a number of reasons. This strengthened the case for regarding the transmission of HIV in the gay community to be a case of self-harm.

Unfortunately, though, matters are murkier than this analysis suggests. The problem is that it is only in the last few years that information about AIDS has been widely available. What does this show? It shows only that prior to, say, 1984 men practicing frequent impersonal anal sex, did not and could not have foreseen the harm they were inflicting on themselves. Hence, they could not consent to it. So the *volenti* maxim does not apply in this case. But it cannot be inferred from this, that the action is no longer a case of self-harm. For it to be a case of one person *wronging* another, that person would have to foresee the harm to the other. But no one in the very early history of AIDS could have known this. Hence, it would be wrong to conclude that those who, in the early years of the disease, infected others, *wronged* them. Now it does not follow from this that in the early years transmission of HIV in the gay community was primarily a self-harm. The morally relevant concept of *consent* needed to distinguish between cases of *self-harm* and *harm to others* cannot be applied until there is a known risk to which people can consent.

This is the situation. When AIDS first surfaced in the gay community no one knew anything about it so they could not have foreseen it. Though many people were infecting others, and in some sense harming them, because they did not and could not foresee the harm they were causing, they did not *wrong* those others. Later, when information was available individuals were harmed, but again not *wronged*, because once the information becomes available to them, they consent to high-risk sex and to the ensuing harm. If this is so, then within the gay community, transmission of HIV falls primarily within the

45

category of *harm to self*. This is not to say that it is always within this domain. Gay men can be raped and they can be deceived about someone's antibody status or about a close partner's philandering.

Collective Harms

Much of the literature on AIDS includes references to alleged harms to others. Quite often those *others* are taken to be a collective. For instance, Ronald Bayer, in a comment on Richard Mohr's thesis about transmission and the private realm, says "Each new carrier of HTLV-lll infection is the potential focus of further social contamination."[37] Dan Beauchamp commences his article "Morality and the Health of the Body Politic" with the statement that "The Acquired Immunodeficiency Syndrome (AIDS) is clearly a public health threat."[38] And C. Everett-Koop in a "Surgeon General's Report on AIDS" admits on the one hand that "No American's life is in danger if he/she or their sexual partners do not engage in high-risk sexual behavior or use shared needles or syringes to inject illicit drugs into the body" but then speaks later of protecting the "health of the nation" and of the American public.[39]

I have argued that within the two highest risk groups AIDS is for the most part a self-inflicted harm and not a harm to others. If this is so, it is unclear how AIDS threatens the public rather than individuals who compose it. After all, it is individuals who get sick and die, not society.

It is obvious how some infectious diseases may be a threat to the public; airborne viruses, for instance, are indiscriminate in who they attack. But AIDS is dramatically unlike these because it is transmitted primarily through cooperative sexual activity: this means that it can be avoided - or put differently, people have some control over whether or not they come into contact with the virus. If most persons with AIDS get the disease through high-risk activity, to which they consent, it is difficult to see how the collective is threatened by it. What, then, can people mean when they say that AIDS is a threat to public health?[40]

A Slippery Concept: Public Health

One way to tackle this question is to reformulate it and ask "What problems are public health problems?" In its infancy public health was concerned mainly with sanitation and the control of infectious disease. It focused narrowly on those health problems which could not be accommodated by individuals themselves. Proper sanitation, for instance, required more than just individual action; it also required a sewage system to which everyone could have access. No single individual could provide this for himself. Public health was originally "limited to measures invoked against nuisances, health hazards with which the individual was powerless to cope".[41]

More recent accounts of *public health* take its scope to be more far-reaching than did its predecessors. Hanlon and Pickett, for instance, claim that "public health must be regarded as an ethical enterprise, as an agent of social change, not just for the sake of change, but to make the *achievement of the improved lot of mankind*".[42]

The main problem with this picture of *public health* is that, according to it almost anything would count as a public health problem.[43] The domain of public health would include everything having to do with the lot of mankind and exclude nothing. AIDS would certainly count as a public health problem, but then so would everything else. This would be unproblematic if it were not the case that matters which are taken to be public health problems are also taken to be open to scrutiny by those who see the health of the public as their mandate. It seems that the notions of 1) a problem for public health authorities and 2) a public health problem, are often wrongly collapsed.

It may be that the distinction between public and private domains has been collapsed in the case of health. Dan Beauchamp, for example, seems to believe that preventable "death and disability" are public goods that should not be subject to the vagaries of the market conception of *justice*. To counter the prevailing individualistic conception of *justice* he advocates what he calls the *public health ethic*. On this topic, he has the following to say

> [T]he central goal of public health should be ethical in nature: The challenging of market-justice as fatally deficient in protecting the health of the public. Further, public health should advocate a *counter-ethic* for protecting the public's health, one articulated in a different tradition of justice and one designed to give the highest priority to minimizing death and disability and to the protection of all human life against the hazards of this world .... the public health ethic is a *counter-ethic* to market-justice and the ethics of individualism as these are applied to the health problems of the public.[44]

Beauchamp's conception of *public health* is a normative one and it is also a departure from how we normally conceive of public health. According to him the mandate of public health is intrinsically ethical. It has moral responsibilities to prevent those diseases and illnesses which can be prevented even if this means redesigning the conception of *justice* which identifies health issues as

48

primarily within the private domain. Beauchamp's proposed *counter-ethic* may be motivated by a desire to insure that preventable illnesses are prevented. But such an extreme measure is not warranted by the goal. Beauchamp's end can be accomplished by providing people with state-funded health care and responsibility for this might go to public health authorities on the grounds that they are best equipped to execute it. There is nothing in this suggestion that requires collapsing 1) and 2). There is no rule which says that *only* health problems which threaten the public are problems to be dealt with by public health authorities. It may be that the underlying reason for conflating the two is the concomitant desire to invoke liberty-limiting policies. If something is a threat to public health, that is, if it harms the public, then government interference may be justified on liberal grounds. To justify such measures, however, it has to be shown that the public is actually harmed; merely asserting that all health problems are public health problems is not going to do the job.

Consider an argument which tries to support the view that HIV/AIDS is a threat to the health of the public. Ronald Bayer seems to be arguing for just this.

The transmission of HTLV-111 has as its first and most obvious consequence a private tragedy: the infection of another human being. But to conceive of such transmission between *consenting adults* as belonging to the private realm alone is a profound mistake (Mohr 1985). Each new carrier of HTLV-111 infection is the potential locus of further social contamination. When few individuals in a community are infected the prospect of undertaking individual and collective measures designed to prevent the spread of AIDS is enhanced. When, however, the levels of infection begin to approach a critical mass, when a level of saturation is approached, the prospect for adopting programs of prophylaxis is diminished.[45]

Bayer has the groundwork for an argument here. He begins by acknowledging that an obvious consequence of the transmission of HIV is the *private tragedy* of infection; then he cautions against construing HIV transmission as belonging solely with the private realm. "Each new carrier of HTLV-111 is the potential locus of further social contamination." Bayer's point is that when AIDS has reached a critical level in society, the possibility of stopping its spread diminishes dramatically. Hence, at a certain point, both individual and collective action will be impotent against the disease.

But this cannot be exactly what Bayer means because when he discusses the high levels of infection in New York and San Francisco, he admits that: "Only the practice of great care in the conduct of one's sexual behavior is left as a mode of protection against infection and reinfection .... the public health challenge is to prevent the replication of New York and San Francisco."[46] One plausible way to read this section is to understand Bayer as identifying New York and San Francisco as places where indeed, infection has reached a critical level. Bayer also acknowledges that cautious sexual behavior remains a mode of protection even in these *infection-saturated* cities. If prevention is possible through individual action and public health authorities can be helpful through education, even in New York and San Francisco, then it is unclear what underlies the notion of a *critical mass*.

The key to this puzzle may lie with the claim that each new HIV positive individual is the "potential locus of further social contamination." But how are we supposed to understand this? How is it that an antibody positive individual could be the potential locus for social contamination? The unwary reader might believe that someone who is HIV positive contaminates society. If so, he is wrong. People who are infected with HIV cannot simply, in virtue of being infected, infect others. HIV is not an airborne virus. Perhaps the expression *social contamination* functions metaphorically. It may mean something like the following: the very presence of AIDS in society contaminates society because it harms the fabric of society. Understood in this way, it makes sense to speak of each new carrier of the virus as the potential locus for social contamination. Society is contaminated not by the virus in a biological sense, but by what it represents metaphorically - AIDS disrupts the fabric of society. Moreover, the more cases of AIDS that there are the more real this disruption becomes. Bayer hints at this as a consequence of AIDS in the following passage:

> The only effective public health strategy for limiting or slowing the further spread of HTLV-111 infection is one that will produce dramatic, perhaps unprecedented changes in the behavior of millions of men and women in this country. Such changes will demand alterations in behaviors that are linked to deep biological and psychological drives and desires. They will demand acts of restraint and even deprivation for extended periods, if not for the lifetimes of those infected and those most at risk for becoming infected.[47]

Bayer is probably right in claiming that a consequence of the AIDS epidemic is that people will have to change their sexual lifestyles if they want to avoid infecting other people and if they want to avoid coming into contact with the virus. But only in a very loose sense of the word *contamination* could this be construed as *social contamination*.

Bayer is also right in thinking that the more cases of AIDS there are, the more difficult it is to avoid the disease because to avoid it one has to avoid coming into contact with partners who have it and that becomes increasingly difficult the more people there are with HIV/AIDS. But it is unclear why this is a problem for society and not for the individual. After all, it is individuals who have to wear condoms and avoid unsafe sex practices.[48] If any behavior is private and in the domain of the individual surely intimate sexual relations are.

What seems to have happened is that there are two competing views of the domain of public health and hence of what will count as a potential problem for it. According to one of these views, anything which pertains to human life is a public health problem. Naturally, on this view, AIDS is a problem for public health officials. In and of itself, this is not problematic. Public health programs may take it upon themselves to provide AIDS awareness literature and to educate people about safe sex practices so that they can determine for themselves how they should conduct their sexual lives. But from the fact that a problem is one that is under the mandate of public health it does not follow that whatever is at issue harms or threatens the public. Nor does it follow that public health authorities ought to do anything to ensure the health of individuals. It may be that those who wish to assign some role to public health with respect to AIDS have felt compelled to justify this role by claiming that those who have AIDS harm society. But this is unnecessary provided that the measures to which public health authorities subscribe do not interfere with individual liberty.

Economic and Social Costs

Society must shoulder the financial burden for the medical care of many of those with HIV/AIDS. In the US 40% of persons with AIDS are covered by Medicaid, a state-funded health insurance program for the poor.[49] The costs of the disease are very high. Estimates of the lifetime costs of treating a person with AIDS in the US range from $50,000 to $60,000.[50] By 1993 the US expects that 450,000 AIDS cases will be diagnosed.[51] Personal medical costs for 1991 are expected to reach between $4.5 and $8.5 billion.

There are also costs associated with AIDS research, education and counselling, HIV testing and hospital precautions, etc. There are costs to people's time, the family, lovers, friends and physicians of persons with AIDS. The time spent with people with AIDS is taken from others; the money spent on AIDS is taken away from other worthy causes.

Showing that there are costs to society because of this epidemic, even showing that these costs are very high and that they constitute a harm, does not show that society is thereby entitled to do *whatever* it wants to do in order to reduce or diminish the harm. To show that liberty-limiting policies can be adopted as a means to diminishing the harm to society caused by AIDS, it would also have to be shown that society has a *claim* on its constituents not to perform actions which will result in this kind of harm to the collective. A corresponding *duty* on the part of individuals to society would also have to be shown to exist.

The kind of action which is causally responsible for the harm to society about which we have been talking is one which contributes to the poor health and death of individuals. Individuals perform actions which result in their illness and death. In turn, illness and death carry with them high costs for society. Do people have a duty to society to remain healthy and thereby reduce the burden on that society? I think not.

It is important to notice about this alleged duty that, if it exists, there is a wide range of behavior and activity to which it would be appropriate to apply it. There are a number of lifestyles which result in illness and death and which also carry with them high medical costs. Smoking and drinking are the most obvious ones. But there are others. High fat diets, stressful occupations, sedentary lifestyles and various forms of the *adventurous life* all contribute to poor health and in some cases death. Now with respect to none of these lifestyles, is it recommended that individuals refrain from them on the grounds that they have a *duty to society* to remain healthy and to keep the costs to society down. If anyone suggested to any of us that we refrain from these activities in order to diminish the burden to society, most of us would regard the suggestion as preposterous and as a wrongful infringement on our liberty. On the other hand, it would not be surprising if people with these very same unhealthy lifestyles were asked to stop them because of duties to family and loved ones.

Why is it that there might be a duty to family to remain in good health, yet not to society in general? This question can be answered by examining more carefully a difference between the two cases. With respect to family, friends and lovers, people have some choice. That is, individuals create families or break them up and walk away from them; and they choose their friends and their lovers. The same is not true with respect to society. Very few people are powerful enough to have any real influence on society and even fewer can pick up their bags and leave when they want to. This difference has an important implication, namely, that with respect to friends, lovers and families, people have an opportunity to choose not only their associations, but also, and in virtue of this, the obligations to which they will be bound. In a sense, giving people the freedom to choose their personal affiliations ensures that they will have a measure of freedom to choose their moral duties. Duties to society are an altogether different matter precisely because people do not have a great deal of freedom with respect to which society they live in. Liberty considerations demand that we be much more parsimonious in the positing of moral duties to society. A proliferation of them would entail a more severe infringement on individual liberty than would a proliferation of moral duties to others.

It is odd that, although in general, no moral duty to remain in good health exists, in the specific case of HIV/AIDS, it is emerging. One cannot help but wonder whether this has more to do with prejudices against the high-risk groups associated with HIV/AIDS than with the existence of a sincere belief that people do have such a duty.

NOTES

1. 'AIDS: A Global Assessment', *Los Angeles Times*, (August (9) 1987), pp. 8-9.

2. Although I think that information about motives and reasons for high-risk behavior is important for answering the second question, I do not go into it in this book.

3. The two questions which I pose here are aligned with two versions of a normative principle which state when, in the *good society*, interference in people's actions is justified. This principle is known as the harm principle. According to the first version, the *strong harm principle*, interference is justified only when the action harms other people (and when interfering will do more good than harm). That is, it is always wrong to interfere with individuals' freedom of action for their own good. This version of the principle corresponds to *hard anti-paternalism*. The second version of the *harm principle*, the *weak harm principle*, states that it is wrong to interfere with a person's self-regarding actions unless those actions are not performed autonomously. This position corresponds roughly, to *soft anti-paternalism*. The difference between the two versions of the principle, as I state them, has mainly to do with the degree of voluntariness required for the action to qualify as one that ought not to be interfered with. My first version of the principle requires that the individual not be coerced and that he or she be competent. My second version states that if an action is not *fully autonomous*, then it can be interfered with. My account of these two versions of the *harm principle* breaks with conventional usage (to the extent that it exists) but does maintain the spirit of an important and traditional distinction. My discussion of this topic has been informed by: Joel Feinberg, *Harm to Self*, Oxford University Press, New York, (1986), (see especially Chapter 17).

4. John Stuart Mill, 'On Liberty', in *John Stuart Mill: On Liberty*, E. Rapaport, ed., (Introduction by E. Rapaport), Hackett Publishing Co., Indianapolis, (1978), p. 73.

5. These arguments will be considered more carefully in Chapter 4.

6. I am grateful to an article written by Richard D. Mohr, 'AIDS, Gays and State Coercion', *Bioethics*, (1987), vol. 1, no. 1, for his insight in formulating the issue in this way.

7. Joel Feinberg, *Harm to Self*, (1986), p. 100.

8. Centers for Disease Control, *AIDS Weekly Surveillance Report*, (March (10) 1985).

9. Lawrence Altman, 'Who's Stricken and How: AIDS Pattern is Shifting', *New York Times*, (February (5) 1989), pp. 1, 28.

10. This intuition is confirmed by the legal view that the intrusion of another agent into the causal chain distinguishes the consequence of the action of one agent from the action of another agent. This is known as the principle of a *novus actus intervenens*. For a discussion of it, see H. L. A. Hart and A. M. Honoree, *Causation in the Law*, Clarendon Press, Oxford, (1959), p. 66, cf. p. 176.

11. I wish to thank Mike Hancock for discussion of this point.

12. Even if people do hold such irrational beliefs it is unclear that we could or should take them into account in forming policy.

13. In this analysis I rely on a consequentialist notion of *moral duty*. Roughly, our moral duties consist of those things which will maximize good consequences. There are, of course, other views about what moral duties we have and about how they ought to be grounded. I adopt a consequentialist framework for identifying moral duties in the case of AIDS because we do not want to establish moral duties that may result in increasing the spread of HIV.

14. For another discussion of *trust*, see Harold Bursztajn, R. T. Feinbloom, R. M. Hamm and A. Brodsky, *Medical Choices, Medical Chances: How Patients, Families and Physicians can Cope with Uncertainty*, Delta/Seymour Lawrence, New York, (1983), pp. 260-92.

15. I wish to thank Harold Wilson and Skip Bassford for helpful comments on this section.

16. John Stuart Mill, 'On Liberty', (1978), p. 79.

17. Dennis Watlington, 'Between the Cracks', *Vanity Fair*, (1987), vol. 50, no. 12, pp. 146, 148.

18. I wish to thank Benjamin Freedman and Eldon Soifer for helpful comments on this section.

19. Don C. Des Jarlais, Samuel R. Friedman and David Strug, 'AIDS and Needle Sharing Within the IV-Drug Use Subculture', in *The Social Dimensions of AIDS: Method and Theory*, D. A. Feldman and T. M. Johnson (eds), Praeger, New York, (1986), p. 113.

20. I do not address the question of what a gay man, who knows that he is HIV positive, ought to do if asked about his antibody status by a potential partner. The answer to this question would seem to depend on whether a duty to tell the truth, under these circumstances, would tend to increase or decrease the practice of safe sex.

21. This does not, of course, commit us to saying that within the drug community, HIV is *always* transmitted by way of self-harm.

22. Richard D. Mohr, 'AIDS, Gays and State Coercion', *Bioethics*, (1987), vol. 1, no. 1, pp. 35-50.

23. There is a great deal of controversy about what constitutes high-risk sex. In this book I take the line that this is a relative concept. Consider the following: Anal sex with a condom is safer than anal sex without a condom; no anal sex would be even safer than anal sex with a condom. Monogamy is safer with a condom than without a condom. Multiple anonymous sex is safer with a condom than without a condom; monogamy with a condom is, in general, safer than multiple anonymous sex with a condom.

24. I do not mean to imply that rape in prisons is primarily among homosexuals. Many men who consider themselves heterosexual and who for the most part are practicing heterosexuals engage in homosexual practices while in prisons.

25. This example should not be construed to mean that infection is likely to occur from one contact with HIV.

26. To avoid this scenario some prisons have adopted a policy of either isolating people who have HIV/AIDS or placing them all in a common area so that they cannot infect those who do not have HIV/AIDS. This policy might result in much greater harm to those who are HIV positive since repeated exposure to the virus may increase one's risk for developing AIDS.

27. Obviously, this is also a moral wrong.

28. From the point of view of policy (when we are trying to decide for a large number of cases and not just particular cases), the only way to identify what is foreseeable is to look at what a hypothetical reasonable person would foresee. I wish to thank Benjamin Freedman for discussion of this point.

29. This does not, of course, preclude the possibility that there are in fact people who would not realize that such an encounter is extremely risky.

What the reasonable person criterion of foreseeability suggests is that they ought to realize this.

30. It may seem odd to impute to gay men a desire for high-risk sex. First of all, I am *not* concerned here with gay men in general, but with those gay men who persist in unsafe sex practices. There are several reasons why gay men might be willing to have unsafe sex, one of which is that they find the risk itself thrilling. This is not as implausible as it may appear to be. Part of the appeal of the *fast track* is that it engenders a more macho stereotype (*Real men want sex*), one which liberates gay men from an effeminate and perhaps oppressive stereotype. Those gay men who endorse this view, of *gay sexuality*, may find safe sex incompatible with it. A concern for safe sex shows an interest in one's health - and might be viewed as betraying an unwillingness to take the risks often associated with the *adventurous man*.

31. I am grateful to Eldon Soifer for this point.

32. Gay writers have responded to this problem with a new crop of novels and stories which depict safe sex in an erotic and exciting way. See, for example, John Preston, ed., *Hot Living: Erotic Stories About Safe Sex*, Alyson Publications, Boston, (1985).

33. Ideally, the question of whether or not gay men expect to be informed of the risk of HIV infection prior to anonymous sexual encounters, would be answered by canvassing gay men and asking them what their expectations are. As far as I know this has not been done. In the absence of such information I can only speculate about what expectations exist among gay men who practice multiple anonymous sex.

34. Of course, this argument would not apply to a monogamous couple, either heterosexual or homosexual, who have agreed to sexual monogamy. This agreement is likely to generate the kinds of expectations about which I have spoken.

35. Since the duty to disclose is a positive duty requiring that one provide information to others, it would seem to entail the additional duty to have the information available. That is, one would have a duty to know one's antibody status.

36. Dreuilhe, for instance, suggests that traditionally impersonal sex in the gay community has served as a way of reducing anxiety: 'Before the epidemic, we often turned to sex to relieve the depression we sometimes felt; there were those who maintained, ten years ago, that an evening in a bathhouse was worth weeks of therapy', Emmanuel Dreuilhe, *Mortal*

Embrace: Living with AIDS, Linda Coverdale Trans. Hill and Wang, New York, (1988), p. 76.

37. Ronald Bayer, 'AIDS, Power and Reason', *The Milbank Quarterly*, (1986), vol. 64 (Suppl. 1), p. 171.

38. Dan E. Beauchamp, 'Morality and the Health of the Body Politic', *Hastings Center Report*, (December 1986), vol. 16, p. 36.

39. C. Everett Koop, 'Surgeon General's Report on Acquired Immune Deficiency Syndrome', *Journal of the American Medical Association*, (November (28) 1986), vol. 256, no. 20, pp. 2784-9.

40. As Richard Mohr points out in 'AIDS, Gays and State Coercion', pp. 46-50, individuals are either healthy or not. The public as a group cannot be healthy or unhealthy except in so far as the individual members of the group are healthy or unhealthy.

41. John J. Hanlon and George E. Pickett, *Public Health: Administration and Practice*, Mosby, St Louis, 8th edition, (1984), p. 4.

42. Ibid.

43. This view of the sphere of *public health* is in keeping with the broad concept of *health* used by the World Health Organization.

44. Dan E. Beauchamp, 'Public Health as Social Justice', in *Moral Problems in Medicine*, R. Macklin and S. Gorovitz (eds), Prentice-Hall, New Jersey, (1983), p. 571.

45. Bayer, 'AIDS, Power and Reason', p. 170-1.

46. Ibid., p. 171.

47. Ibid., p. 170.

48. Even if this is a consequence of HIV/AIDS, it is not an unequivocally bad consequence. Many gay men report that their relationships have improved as a result of the epidemic. Although they find that they have yet to master the skills needed to develop long-term intimacies, they value such relationships and the opportunity to cultivate them.

49. Harvey V. Fineberg, 'The Social Dimensions of AIDS', *Scientific American*, (October 1988), vol. 259, no. 4, p. 132.

50. Ibid., p. 133.

51. Ibid.

3
Sex, Drugs and Autonomy

On the basis of the last chapter those who endorse the *strong harm principle* would urge that no liberty-limiting social policy is justified in the case of AIDS since, for the most part, the harm that is experienced by gay men and IV drug-users is a self-inflicted one.[1] Gay men who engage in high-risk sexual activity consent to do so.[2] Adult IV drug-users may also be construed as consenting to an activity which they know to be dangerous and which they know may cause them harm. They are not grabbed by the arm and forced to inject narcotics into their veins using needles which have been used by others.

Yet the *strong harm principle* does not exhaust the possible grounds for interfering with basically self-regarding actions in the *good society*. Because it might be the case that the risky actions of gay men and IV drug-users are not performed autonomously it is open to those who endorse the *weak harm principle* to reintroduce the possibility of liberty-limiting social policy. I shall argue, however, that even according to the *weak harm principle* liberty-limiting social policy is not justified.

There is good reason to think that, for the most part, the high-risk behavior of IV-users and gay men is not autonomous, for reasons which have to do with society and not with them. Because, in this case, autonomy is diminished by social conditions, I argue that how society ought to respond will be different from how it ought to respond if the source of the problem were some feature, say biological, of those in the high-risk groups. If this analysis is right, then AIDS prevention measures which would further interfere with the autonomy of gay men and IV drug-users are morally unacceptable. To see where the *weak harm principle* stands on this issue more information is needed, namely, information about whether or not the high-risk actions of gay men and IV drug-users are performed autonomously.

Autonomy and Liberty

Autonomy

Because according to the *weak harm principle* autonomy figures importantly in the evaluation of AIDS policy, an understanding of the concept of *autonomy* is required. According to the view that I shall use, autonomous individuals are self-directed.[3] They act in accordance with the desires which they have come to endorse. Gerald Dworkin has the following to say about this view of autonomy.

It is the attitude a person takes towards the influences motivating him which determines whether or not they are to be considered *his*. Does he identify with them, assimilate them to himself, view himself as the kind of person who wishes to be motivated in these particular ways? If, on the contrary, a man resents his being motivated in certain ways, is alienated from those influences, resents acting in accordance with them, would prefer to be the kind of person who is motivated in different ways, then those influences, even though they may be causally effective, are not viewed as *his*.[4]

Thus the actions of autonomous agents are expressions of their second-order desires (second-order desires have as their object first-order desires). For example, a cigarette smoker who is trying to quit smoking, may have a second-order desire not to smoke, and a very strong first-order desire to smoke. This smoker does not smoke autonomously. With autonomous persons there is a symmetry between how they act and how they want to act. They are not driven to act by desires with which they do not identify. An autonomous smoker is one who has both first and second-order desires to smoke. He may, for instance, see smoking as an expression of his carefully cultivated overwrought and anxiety-ridden persona.

The idea that people can be motivated to act on the basis of desires which are unauthentic should be kept in mind because it may be that the desires responsible for much of the high-risk behavior of gay men and IV drug-users are unauthentic. To say that gay men and IV drug-users act on the basis of unauthentic desires and hence do not act autonomously is *not* to say or to imply that everyone else does act autonomously. That is, in saying that gay men who choose the *fast track* do not do so autonomously, I am not saying, for example, that heterosexuals who choose monogamy are acting autonomously.[5] The psychological notion of an *adaptive preference* is important in explaining

why it is plausible to say that the behavior that puts gay
men and IV drug-users at high risk for HIV/AIDS is not
autonomous.

The hunch behind this crucial concept is that some
desires and preferences are shaped by the feasible set of
options open to people, that is, by the context. People
come to have preferences and desires as a way of reducing
cognitive dissonance.[6] Put differently, if a person desires
something which he cannot have because, for whatever
reason, it is not available to him, in order to decrease the
unhappiness associated with the frustrated desire, he may
come to have a desire which he can satisfy. The latter is
an *adaptive preference*. For example, women who were
denied opportunities to pursue rewarding careers outside
of the home may have cultivated very strong desires for
domestic bliss simply because these desires could be
satisfied while the others would only lead to frustration
and unhappiness.

Someone who acts on the basis of an adaptive preference
often does not act autonomously because the desire that is
causally efficacious is externally generated. The contented
housewife of my example, craves domesticity not because
it reflects who she is, but because desires to do otherwise,
in a society which thwarts them, carry with them too much
pain.[7]

There is another moral to be drawn from this story,
namely, that society, specifically by way of the options it
makes available to people, may be causally responsible for
the desires which people come to have. The contented
housewife's desire for domestic bliss is socially induced;
she might well have other desires were it not for the fact
that society is arranged in such a way that those desires
are not likely to be satisfied. Policy-makers ought to bear
in mind that the desires and wants that people have may

be a function not so much of what they really want, but of the options that are made available to them.[8]

Autonomy can also be reduced through *psychological oppression*. Sandra Bartky defines this important concept in the following way:

> To be psychologically oppressed is to be weighed down in your mind; it is to have a harsh dominion exercised over your self-esteem. The psychologically oppressed become to themselves their own oppressors; they come to exercise harsh dominion over their own self-esteem. Differently put, psychological oppression can be regarded as the "internalization of intimations of inferiority".[9]

Psychological oppression is in one sense self-imposed. Individuals who believe of themselves that they are not fully autonomous agents may also become their own oppressors. Women, for instance, who have internalized the view that they are capable only of being cute and amusing may come to believe this of themselves and act accordingly. Ante-bellum blacks who accepted the view that they were less than fully rational human beings chose not to exercise those capacities which we associate with self-determining agents, and thus we had the *Uncle Tom*.[10]

To enhance individual autonomy two avenues are open. First, positive steps can be taken to ensure that individuals have the personal wherewithal to come to know themselves and to formulate desires in keeping with their *true self*. A society committed to individual autonomy might well provide universal access to psychotherapy. Second, to ensure that individuals can cultivate authentic desires and then act in accordance with them, restrictions which might inhibit the formulation of such desires need to be removed. Making a wide range of significant options available to people will give them a genuine opportunity to develop and evaluate desires to see which are authentic to them. It is at this junction that *autonomy* and *liberty* meet.

Liberty

The notion of *autonomy* endorsed here is a strong one; it requires of the individual that he be self-aware and that he act in ways which he has come to identify as constituting his self. To respect autonomy in this sense, society must give individuals extensive liberty so that a) they may explore different conceptions of the *good life* and b) they may act on the conceptions which they favor. To make practically possible a pluralism of different conceptions of the *good life* and an exploration of these, individuals require in addition to liberty of action an arena of privacy. For people to feel free enough to experiment with different conceptions of the *good life*, privacy is absolutely necessary. In the service of autonomy, individuals must be provided with privacy and liberty of action.

According to the value that the *weak harm principle* places on autonomous decision-making, it is important that any action taken by government be such that it preserve as much as possible individual claims to self-determination and autonomy. In practice, this means that society has a duty not to interfere, by way of policy and legal measures, with the autonomous and self-regarding actions of individuals.[11] In view of this, measures designed to halt the spread of HIV/AIDS must be evaluated with a critical eye. This is not to say that the non-autonomous individual ought necessarily to be interfered with. The goal is to reinstate autonomous decision-making. How best to achieve this end depends very much on what the conditions are which impede autonomy.

The idea underlying the *weak harm principle* is that a person is not protected from himself when he is prevented from acting in ways which are not fully autonomous. If the conduct is not autonomous, then it does not really reflect the person; that is, in some sense it is not really his action.[12] This position, if correct, would seem to have serious implications for AIDS social policy. If high-risk behavior among gay men and IV-users is not fully autonomous then apparently on this view, it is open to interference.

Autonomy and High-Risk Behavior

Because the concern here is with AIDS social policy, the focus is not on particular actions, but on a class of actions. The goal is to find out if, in general, the high-risk behavior of those in the two highest risk groups for HIV/AIDS are performed autonomously. Determining whether or not an action is autonomous is not an easy task at the best of times, and it is not made any easier when the focus is on a class of actions. My strategy will be to look at what sociological and psychological research on gay men and IV-users has to offer - to see what explanations are given of high-risk behavior. An exhaustive analysis of the degree of autonomy involved in high-risk actions cannot be hoped for, but a step in that direction can be taken by considering these actions in the light of three obstacles to autonomy: incompetency, coercion and ignorance.[13]

Before turning to questions about autonomy and high-risk behavior, it will be helpful to look at what specific actions are high risk. Identifying behavior which is associated with the sexual life of gay men (i.e. anal receptive sex, multiple anonymous partners) as high-risk sex, is a controversial matter.[14]

The idea of *safe sex* which prevailed during the early and mid-eighties has more recently been replaced with that of *safer sex*. This change implies that sex is not entirely safe, that there are degrees of safety. Many people (especially within the gay community) maintain that sex (including anal receptive sex) with a condom is safe.[15] Obviously, anal sex is safer with a condom than without one. But it is equally obvious that in addition to condom use, it would be even safer to refrain altogether from anal sex and to cut down drastically the number of sexual partners one has unless one practices only frottage.[16] Epidemiologists William Heyward and James Curran from the Centers for Disease Control have recently confirmed this.

In the US most sexual transmission of HIV has been among homosexual men. The risk of infection in these men increases with the number of sexual partners and the frequency with which they are the receptive partner in anal intercourse. The insertive partner in anal intercourse, however, has also been known to become infected with HIV....[17]

In my discussion of high risk choices among gay men, I focus on frequent impersonal sex as a risky practice. I do this, in part, because the questions asked need to be answered by looking retrospectively at the gay community. Most gay men who now have HIV/AIDS acquired it long before either safe or safer sex became prominent notions - when information about what constitutes these was foggy. To find out whether the behavior that put both gay men and IV-users at increased risk for infection was performed autonomously, we have to look at what the members of these communities were doing and why they were doing it when they became infected. Frequent impersonal anal sex was central to the sexual lives of many gay men.

Competency and Incompetency

For a choice to be autonomous the chooser must, at the very least, be competent to make it. A minimal requirement for competency is that individuals have the requisite intellectual skills to assess an action and its consequences and to perform simple means/end reasoning.[18] Competency is not an all or nothing state of affairs. Individuals may be competent to make some decisions, but not others.[19] For instance, some elderly people have been found to be incompetent to manage their own financial affairs, though perfectly capable of managing their other personal affairs. In the case at hand, the following question needs to be answered. Are individuals who put themselves at risk for HIV/AIDS competent to choose the actions which place them at high risk?

To some, the decision to risk coming into contact with HIV/AIDS constitutes *prima facie* evidence of the chooser's incompetence. The reasoning goes like this. AIDS is a fatal disease with a frequently painful death. Anyone who would choose to put themselves at risk for it is insane and hence incompetent. At least one of the assumptions here is true, namely, that people who are insane are not competent decision-makers. But even the insane are competent to make some decisions. For instance, they are competent to choose vanilla over chocolate ice cream.

This *anyone who would do that* argument suffers from a couple of problems. Consideration of the content of a decision alone is not enough to establish that its chooser is incompetent. It certainly could not show that an individual is incompetent in a global sense and it is highly unlikely that it could show that he is incompetent with respect to specific matters. Normally, some insight into the reasons for the decision is necessary before competency can be judged. Consider the following example. Imagine that Tom informs us that he will cut off his right foot because he has a callous that has been irritating him. Tom's choice suggests insanity in so far as his goal, to put an end to the irritation caused by the callous, does not justify his means, chopping off his right foot. But knowing only that Tom has decided to eliminate an offensive foot is not enough to let us know that he is incompetent for there are circumstances under which this would be perfectly reasonable. Tom's foot might be gangrenous, for example.

Similarly, a number of plausible reasons could be given by gay men for some of their high-risk choices. The desire for bathhouse sex might be accounted for on the basis of a strong preference for impersonal sex in public or simply a preference for risky sex. IV-users place themselves at risk through the sharing of needles. They might give the following reasons for their choice: a desire for a sense of collegiality, a desire to maximize needle-use because needles are a scarce commodity, or a desire to minimize the legal repercussions of being found in possession of a needle. For both high-risk groups, a variety of reasons can be identified that go toward explaining why high-risk choices are made. In neither case is it necessary to seriously question the capacity for means/end judgments.

Still, one might insist that with respect to both IV drug-users and gay men with risky lives, the choice of the goal, or the goal itself, betrays a lack of competency. It is difficult to see why this is so. Choosers who put themselves at risk for HIV/AIDS probably do not have as their end to put themselves at risk for AIDS. Rather, high-risk activities are a means to other desired ends: impersonal sex, a sense of collegiality, avoidance of legal repercussions. Some of these ends might be ones which many people do not particularly value, but that is not the same as showing that they are irrational. Countless numbers of persons frequently seek just these ends and few people think to query their competency. Heterosexual men and women seek impersonal sex at singles bars; clubs and organizations of various kinds provide people with a sense of collegiality; and tax evaders, jaywalkers and drunk drivers go out of their way to avoid the hand of the law.

If the goals themselves do not betray incompetency and the combination of the goals and the means used to achieve them fail to reveal it, there is little reason to suppose that there is anything to the argument that to choose high-risk behavior is to be incompetent. So, a blanket ascription of incompetency simply on the basis of a high-risk choice cannot be made. This conclusion corresponds to our intuitions about other high-risk choices. We are not tempted to describe those with a preference for high-risk activities such as car racing, hang gliding and sky diving as incompetent simply because they opt for these high-risk pleasures. Personal repulsion for certain sorts of activities should not be allowed to stand as a serious objection to what are perceived as distasteful lifestyles.

The crux of the *anyone who would do that* argument is not high-risk activities *per se*, because it is limited to particular high-risk activities - those, no doubt, which the objector does not believe are worth the risk. But this is obviously a matter of personal taste. There are no *per se* risks which are worthwhile. Whether or not a risk is worth that which is risked depends on the values, goals and desires of the person taking it.

Although universal incompetence cannot be assigned to those who choose high-risk activities, it might still be argued that some people who develop AIDS are incompetent. What about adults who are addicted to narcotics? Surely, when drug-addicts are under the pressure of withdrawal, they are incompetent and because of this fail to make autonomous choices to assume the high-risk activity of sharing works.

There may be something to this objection, but it is not clear that what is at issue is the individual's competency or that it can be assumed simply from the fact that someone is addicted to narcotics that it thereby follows that he is incompetent to make judgments about whether or not he wants to use the injection equipment which has been used by others. There is no reason to think that a desire, even a very strong desire for a narcotic, has the effect of impairing one's reasoning faculties. A desire, if it is strong enough, may override one's judgment, or may override one's desire to make use of one's capacities for judgment. But this sort of thing happens all the time and when it does, most people are not inclined to conclude that the individuals concerned are incompetent.[20]

Consider the following scenario. Smith, who is overcome with passion and desire for Brown, betrays her husband and begins an adulterous affair. Her desire for Brown overrides her judgment (in fact judgment may not enter into her calculations at all), but most of us are not tempted to conclude from this that she is incompetent to judge. Rather, we conclude either that she decided that lust should trump reason, or that she suffers from weakness of the will. In any case, we do not conclude that she is incompetent to choose in favor of Brown simply because she has a strong desire for him or because she has a desire which she cannot resist. That we do not think her incompetent is borne out by the fact that neither we, nor Mr Smith for that matter, would be willing to excuse her on the grounds that she is incompetent. She is taken to be responsible for her actions.

There is another reason why it would be a mistake to assume that adults addicted to narcotics are incompetent to make high-risk choices. Even if it is assumed, contrary to the above argument, that, once addicted to narcotics, individuals do not choose or act competently, it would not follow from this that their initial choice to inject narcotics and to become addicts is not a competent one.[21] That is, at some point individuals who do not yet have a strong desire for narcotics make a decision to take them.[22] There is no reason to think that at that point they are incompetent unless, of course, one falls back on the argument that anyone who chooses high-risk activities is incompetent. But I have already shown that this argument is inadequate.

The arguments which might be advanced to undermine the competency of gay men and IV drug-users to choose high-risk activities do not work. It cannot be concluded on this ground alone that their high-risk choices are not made autonomously.[23] This point needs to be underscored. Of the three categories being looked at to assess whether or not gay men and IV drug-users are making autonomous high-risk choices, competency is the only one which has to do exclusively with them as individuals and hence the only one that could clearly justify limiting their liberty. The other two, coercion and ignorance, have much more to do with external conditions than internal ones. If there is an obstacle to autonomy as a result of either of these two conditions, then the chances are that some change to the external conditions is warranted.

Coercion and Manipulation

Coercion can also interfere with the autonomy of a choice. A paradigm case of a coerced choice is the *your money or your life* threat. A man who hands over his wallet at gunpoint does not make an autonomous choice to do so. He is forced to do so because the alternative to not turning over the money represents a far greater harm than what is demanded.

The psychological analogue of coercion is manipulation. People can be manipulated into making certain choices and not others. Adaptive preference formation is a good example of this; by drastically reducing the number of significant options open to people they are manipulated into formulating certain desires. Both coercion and manipulation can interfere with autonomous decision-making. And it should not be assumed that only individuals are capable of manipulating and coercing others. Society and institutions can do so by reducing the options open to individuals.

Is there any reason to think that the high-risk choices made by those in the two high-risk groups for HIV/AIDS are coerced because of reduced options? A close look at the context in which high-risk activities are chosen by gay men and IV drug-users suggests that the answer is yes.

Gay Men
Frequent impersonal anal sex turned out to be very dangerous for gay men. I am not going to look at why gay men have anal sex as I assume this can be explained on the basis of the pleasure that they derive from it. The same simple explanation does not obviously hold with respect to multiple anonymous sexual encounters. It is by no means clear why many anonymous partners are more desirable than one familiar partner. This is especially

mysterious in view of the standing assumption that people desire the kind of intimacy, trust and security that are often associated with long-term relationships.

One way to find out why frequent, impersonal sex has become central to *gay sex* is to look at what makes it desirable from the point of view of gay men.[24] Gay bathhouses are one of the primary venues for anonymous sexual encounters. Alan Bell and Martin Weinberg give the following account of the appeal of the bathhouses.

> The major function of the gay bath is to provide an inexpensive place where homosexual men can engage in frequent, anonymous sexual activity without fear of social or legal reprisal.... The cost was low, much cheaper than a motel room, and a patron might have nearly a dozen sexual encounters while he was there.[25]

In another paper which examines the success of the baths from the point of view of the men attending them, the following concern was voiced.

> Male participants are often concerned about sanctions and dangers. Thus ideal conditions include features that protect the participant - e.g. a safe setting with low public visibility....[26]

Together these remarks show that, at least in part, gay men go to the baths because the baths are protected sanctuaries where they can safely pursue sex with other men. In turn, the desire for a safe place for sex can be explained by prevailing social attitudes to homosexuality. If the public celebrated homosexual liaisons in the same way it does heterosexual ones, gay men would have no reason to desire a safe setting for their sexual life. Homosexual displays of affection and sexuality would be viewed with the same benevolent eye as heterosexual ones. The desire for anonymous sexual trysts can also be explained by social conditions. Sex with unknown others is one way to ensure that one's sexual proclivities remain unknown.

It would be a mistake to think that all gay men with a desire for frequent impersonal sexual encounters have this desire for the same reason. A few alternatives need to be considered. Three main reasons for preferring impersonal to personal sex come to mind. 1) Impersonal sex may be desirable in and of itself. That is, there may be some aspect of it which is itself sexually gratifying and which is sought for its own sake. 2) Impersonal sex may have symbolic importance. 3) Impersonal sex might be a last resort in a world of diminished options.

Consider the first reason. In the following passage, from an autobiographical novel of John Rechy's entitled *The Sexual Outlaw*, the intrinsic value of impersonal sex is illuminated.

> Each moment of his outlaw existence [the sexual outlaw] confronts repressive laws, repressive *morality*. Parks, alleys, subways, tunnels, garages, streets - these are the battlefields. To the sex hunt he brings a sense of choreography, ritual, and mystery - sex - cruising with an electrified instinct that sends and receives messages of orgy at any moment, any place.[27]

For Rechy's *outlaw* there is a thrill to impersonal sex which is associated with its social taboo. It provides the *outlaw* with something that he cannot obtain from a more orthodox sexual life. Still, it is important to remember that we are dealing with desires here and that they are not immune to outside influences. The Rechy passage suggests that the *outlaw*'s desire for impersonal sex is intimately connected with the fact that it is forbidden. If so, and if the *outlaw* is unaware of this influence or, though aware, does not endorse it, then he fails to act autonomously. His desire for *the hunt* is largely motivated by an external influence - repressive morality.

Now consider the second reason, that impersonal sex has symbolic and political significance. In *The Plague Years*, David Black suggests that for gay men impersonal sex represents liberation from an effeminate and basically passive stereotype. There is certainly an element of this in the above Rechy quotation. The term used to denote the one who cruises, *outlaw*, connotes an image of a strong, virile, macho character. Black speaks of the significance of impersonal sex for the gay community in the following passage.

> If fast-track gays ... saw themselves as pioneers, like pioneers, they had to be tough. What they wanted was sex, not love ... American homosexuals were cultivating the macho stereotype - the biker-lumberjack-Hemingway tough guy - that straight men, under the influence of feminism, were abandoning. Giving up promiscuous sex meant giving up a hard-won *positive* identity, going back to the Nellie stereotype....[28]

For some men, then, frequent impersonal sex has come to represent liberation from an oppressive stereotype. The *fast track* was seen by many gay men as a mechanism through which they could transcend the *sissy* stereotype and adopt a new one. According to this latter, they were no longer passive and impotent victims of society but strong men with whom society would have to contend. On this explanation, the appeal of frequent impersonal sex is tied to the gay community vis-a-vis mainstream society; it is a reaction to a fundamentally anti-gay society. In other words, some gay men turned to frequent impersonal sex in response to the pressure of social discrimination and stereotyping. Had society not discriminated, the need for liberation would not have existed. It is also worth mentioning that on this explanation a few anonymous sexual encounters are not sufficient to achieve the macho stereotype of which Black speaks. As we all know *Real Men want sex and lots of it.*

Third, those who seek impersonal sex may do so because of reduced options. Society, even contemporary society, discriminates against homosexuals. Gay men and women remain a deviant sub-culture within mainstream society; the usual channels for achieving personal sex within long-term relationships are closed to them. Because of this, some men may view impersonal sex as "a catalyst in the development of a more personal relationship".[29] Others may regard it as the primary option open to them in a society which condemns homosexuality. This view receives some support from Bell and Weinberg.

[O]ur data tend to belie the notion that homosexual affairs are apt to be inferior imitations of heterosexuals' premarital or marital involvements. The fact that homosexual liaisons, unlike those of their heterosexual counterparts, are not encouraged or legally sanctioned by society probably accounts for their relative instability.... Our data indicate that a relatively steady relationship with a love partner is a very meaningful event in the life of a homo-sexual man or woman.... In any case, most of our homosexual respondents spoke of these special relationships in positive terms and clearly were not content to limit their sexual contacts to impersonal sex.[30]

Those who practice impersonal sex either as a means to achieving personal sex in a society which discriminates against them, or because of reduced options, do not do so with full autonomy. The options open to gay men are reduced by society through discriminatory legislation and harsh attitudes to homosexuality. Because of this, the choices that they do make are coerced; gay men might well choose a long-term partner were that a real option.

It might be argued that surely if gay men wanted something other than multiple anonymous sex, they would voice this desire. As a matter of fact, they have done the opposite. Some gay theorists rigorously defend the *fast track* and among gay men there is strong support for this position. It is surely implausible to argue that the desire for multiple anonymous sexual encounters is not autonomous.

That gay men desire and defend the *fast track* can be explained by invoking the concepts of *adaptive preference* and of *psychological oppression*. Adaptive desires are not desired any less because of their genesis; they may be just as strong as non-adaptive ones. Gay men who have come to desire frequent anonymous sex because there is no real option to it, desire it just as much as if it were an autonomous desire. Furthermore, the phenomenon of psychological oppression can account for the fact that this lifestyle is vigorously defended. Those who have been oppressed often identify with their oppressors, and in turn, come to oppress themselves. If, on top of this, they are smart and imaginative, the mechanisms by which they oppress themselves may be quite sophisticated. Put differently, it is not at all surprising that gay man have constructed elaborate theories in defence of their social and sexual mores.

IV Drug-Users

IV drug-users do not fare much better with respect to autonomy, and more specifically, manipulation, than gay men. To see whether those who share needles do so autonomously, the reasons for participating in this high-risk activity will have to be examined. If there are social conditions which mandate needle-sharing in the drug community, then to that extent the high-risk behavior of IV-users is coerced and unlikely to be autonomous. According to Des Jarlais, Friedman and Strug, there are three contexts in which needles are shared: as an initiation rite, with running partners and in shooting galleries.[31]

Initiating people into the world of injected drugs is called *giving them their wings*. It has been described as *exciting*, *dangerous* and *romantic*. In the following description a young man describes the excitement and peer identification associated with the experience.

> I used to watch Jim shoot up, and I became very curious about the rush and the high. So one night, I was alone with Jim and Tom and before I knew it, Jim was preparing the dope, and Tom was holding my arm. I was excited. My best friend's older brother was *giving me my wings*.... Jim inserted the number 25 needle into my arm. He got a fast hit, and I went flying off into heaven. Ooh, It was nice and euphoric. I fell in love with heroin that night in my good friend's house. I felt very secure. Like I wasn't alone any more. I realized that things wouldn't be the same for me, now that I've used the needle.[32]

Although the man who is *getting his wings* is surprised at the event, his remarks also show that he had been flirting with the idea of injected drugs for some time.[33] Through the initiation, the two participants become good friends, providing each other with a sense of security and freedom from loneliness. Nothing in the initiate's remarks suggest coercion, or even undue pressure. There is not even a hint of dissatisfaction with the decision. The high-risk activity seems to be embraced for its own sake; it is itself thrilling and exciting. To introduce into this scenario one's own needle might detract from the impulsive, romantic and exciting tone which is sought in the event.

Needle-sharing does, however, seem to be less than fully autonomous in the other two main contexts. Consider the case of *running partners*. Because IV drug-use is illegal, along with the activities associated with it (theft, prostitution), many addicts team up as a more efficient way of achieving their ends. *Running partners* "scheme, hustle, and boost" together as well as "get off" together.[34] The relationship is one of teamwork and cooperation and acts as a substitute family. Cooperation extends to needle-sharing because "needles are in short supply, and withdrawal creates a sense of urgency."[35]

Of course, needles would not be in short supply and withdrawal would not present an imperative if narcotics were not illegal. Similarly, there would not be a need for a running partner if there were nothing to run after. In this case then, the sharing of needles is intimately connected with the way that society is organized. When narcotic use is prohibited, individuals who want to take drugs must do so at high risk to themselves. To secure narcotics they must team up and to avoid the pain of involuntary withdrawal from narcotics, which is often a function of the cost and scarcity of them, they must make use of whatever injection equipment is available.

Consider the third context in which needles are shared, *shooting galleries*. These represent by far the greatest risk of HIV/AIDS for IV drug-users. Shooting galleries are places where, for a fee, individuals can rent the equipment needed to inject drugs and the services of someone to assist them if required. Unused needles are available, but at twice the cost of used ones. A needle might be shared by any number of people. People choose to inject drugs in these very high-risk locations because of the circumstances in which narcotics must be purchased and used. In their study, Des Jarlais, Friedman and Strug explain why shooting galleries are used.

- Galleries provide the privacy and equipment needed for injecting drugs.
- Galleries are usually located in close proximity to purchasing areas. This is important because of the pressure of withdrawal and the need for quick recourse to dealers.
- Galleries provide a forum in which IV drug-users may interact socially and may obtain valuable information about drug sources and police activities.
- Galleries, because they rent out the necessary equipment, reduce the risk of arrest which one incurs by carrying needles. (AIDS has increased reluctance to carry one's own needle because IV-users now fear stronger police reprisal in case a needle should prick an officer.)[36]

IV-users have certain practical needs which arise because narcotics are illegal. For example, if heroin were not illegal, involuntary withdrawal would not be a problem. Addicts would have easy access to both narcotics and injecting equipment. The crux of the matter is that shooting galleries would no longer serve a useful purpose if narcotics could be obtained legally.

The high-risk behavior of IV drug-users is like that of gay men in so far as much of it is a consequence of social factors. Because the activities that IV-users engage in are illegal, they are *forced* to perform these activities in ways that ultimately endanger their lives.

Some people may urge that *forced* is an inappropriate choice of words. IV-users perform activities which are illegal; they choose to endanger their own lives indirectly by choosing to act illegally. The assumption here is that society is justified in making narcotic use illegal. But this is far from clear. Narcotic use, like alcohol use, is a self-regarding action; the consequences fall mainly on those who use illicit substances. Intervention in this case is paternalistic and the burden is on those who want to intervene to show that it is justified.[37] IV-users who choose to act contrary to the law may be acting contrary to an unjust law.

Ignorance

A lack of relevant information about an action or its consequences can reduce the autonomy of the act. For example, a patient who lacks relevant information concerning alternative therapies cannot make an informed choice about what course to follow. A choice made without relevant information is not fully autonomous. Individuals who are unaware of exactly what they are choosing are not, to say the least, in an ideal position to fully endorse the choice.

Gay Men

There has been widespread press coverage of HIV/AIDS since the mid-eighties. In fact, there have been complaints that the press were excessively zealous in their coverage of this disease. Headlines such as the one that appeared on the cover of *Life* magazine, "Now No One is Safe from AIDS" do not speak well for them.[38] In addition to the coverage HIV/AIDS has received in the mainstream press, governments, educators and community organizations have distributed AIDS awareness literature and campaigned on behalf of safe sex education. Mainly, the focus has been on heterosexuals and adolescents.

Still, what is true of the mid-eighties was not true when people first come into contact with the virus in the mid to late seventies. People could not have had information about something for which no information existed. The first persons with HIV/AIDS acted out of ignorance. They did not know that what are now characterized as high-risk activities were high-risk activities.

What about the early eighties? Consider the baths again. Did people, frequenting the baths, know the extent of the danger they faced there? Was their choice to go to the baths and participate in high-risk sexual activity an informed one? San Francisco, though by no means paradigmatic, is a good example. There, gay men constitute a strong, well-organized, politically powerful and sophisticated group. If there is a place where the gay community would have been well informed, it would have been in San Francisco.

Frances Fitzgerald, in an excellent article for the *New Yorker*, untangles the web of controversy concerning the San Francisco baths.[39] The question of whether or not to regulate them became a highly political one in San Francisco, with different interest groups taking different stands, and others simply passing the responsibility on; for some, there was a strong interest in shielding the gay community from the facts about AIDS.

By 1984 San Francisco had the highest number of AIDS cases per capita in the US. A 1985 survey showed that 50% of gay men in San Francisco had been exposed to HIV. AIDS struck at the heart of the San Francisco gay community. Although the press had shown that the virus was transmitted through sexual contact involving bodily fluids, a 1983 study conducted by Leon McKusick showed that only 30% of gay men in San Francisco had changed their sexual behavior because of AIDS. Most gay men had not taken the threat seriously enough. Some even claimed to have increased their participation in high-risk sex.[40]

This comes as a surprise given the amount of coverage that AIDS had apparently received. Responsibility for disseminating information about the transmission of the virus lay with the San Francisco Health Department, but apparently they had been less than successful in conveying information about AIDS to gay men. The literature distributed by the Health Department was aimed at informing the general public that AIDS was not contagious and could not be transmitted through casual contact. No literature had appeared in city clinics frequented by gay men and the gay community had done little in the way of warning men of the dangers of high-risk sex. There is, unfortunately, also evidence that some members of the gay community were interested in suppressing information about the magnitude of the problem in San Francisco. Consider the following. The findings of the University of California Medical Center report on the incidence of AIDS in the Castro had been published in the *San Francisco Chronicle*.[41] However, just before the article appeared, a number of gay activists requested that the report be suppressed because its findings would hurt business in the Castro district and would reduce the chances of a gay rights bill passing in Sacramento.[42] With respect to the literature that did appear there were complaints. One spokesperson for the gay community had the following to say:

"The educational program is crap ... Look at the new AIDS Foundation posters. There's one with a photograph of two sexy naked men with their asses turned to the camera, and underneath there's a message about the joys of safe sex. Look, I've seen a lot of men with Kaposi's sarcoma. It's a hideous, disfiguring disease. A Hollywood make-up man couldn't duplicate it. There should be pictures of it. But the gay press has never carried a picture, and when *Time* and *Newsweek* did stories on AIDS the worst they showed were the lesions on a leg".[43]

The first literature that emerged from the San Francisco Health Department was equally mild: "Limit your use of recreational drugs" and "Enjoy more time with fewer partners" was the proffered advice.[44] Clearly, the information that reached gay men living in San Francisco in 1983 was not designed to maximize information about AIDS.

Now there may be moral reasons for exercising restraint on the distribution of information. Objections to paternalistic intervention apply equally well to information as to actions. Forcing someone to read literature which he doesn't want to read for his own good violates his claims to autonomy.[45] If someone doesn't want to know about the danger connected with high-risk sexual activity, it would be wrong to force him to.

The merits of this argument are unclear, but in any event, it does not seem to apply to the case at hand. There is no indication that individual members of the gay community have a desire not to have information about AIDS. Nor is it unreasonable to suppose that most gay men would want information relevant to their health maintenance. Perhaps the *thrill seekers*, those interested in high-risk sex for its own sake, do not want to know anything about the gory details of AIDS. But it is just as reasonable to suppose that their pleasure would be enhanced if they discovered that the risk is greater than they first thought and hence that they would prefer more information to less. Even if some individuals would rather have less information, there is no reason to think that merely making information available to them is tantamount to forcing them to peruse it. They are still free to turn away from whatever is made available.

It was in a politically confused climate that the controversy about the baths arose. There were some in the gay community who believed that both regulation and closing the baths was a direct assault on the hard won civil liberties of gay men and there were others who believed that the baths were killing gay men. But few of these people were disinterested. Bathhouses were a highly profitable business in San Francisco. They were frequented by local residents and were a strong attraction for tourists. On the other side, there was pressure to close them, but that could be explained by a growing panic against gay men. Furthermore, many believed that closing them might lead to a gay backlash, and this in turn could destroy political careers. It is also worth pointing out that many gay men and IV drug-users did not have much confidence in the veracity of the information that they were getting from the media. On the basis of past experience neither group had reason to trust the medical community or mainstream press. Dreuilhe voices this view in the following passage:

> At a time when the first few hundred victims had already fallen, most drug addicts and homosexuals suspected the authorities of trying to interfere with their personal liberties by concocting a new disease out of thin air.[46]

The point to be gleaned from this is that even as late as 1983 in a city as politicized as San Francisco, the information that was reaching the gay community was not sufficient to allow individual men to make fully informed choices about high-risk activities. A number of people had an interest in maintaining San Francisco as a high profile gay haven and hence an interest in underplaying the threat that high-risk sexual activity posed to gay men. Although one cannot prove that there is a causal connection between the two, it would seem that a consequence of the activities of these rival factions in the early eighties in San Francisco was a reduction in the amount and quality of information that gay men had available to them, and that this, in turn, meant that gay men were taking risks they might otherwise not have taken.

Proof of a causal connection cannot be given here. There is, though, convincing evidence that had gay men been given more information, they would have reduced their risk taking activities. In a study headed by Leon McKusick which was conducted in San Francisco, it was shown that there were substantial changes in the sexual behavior of gay men with respect to persons other than their primary partners.

The AIDS epidemic has precipitated fundamental changes in the sex lives of gay men in San Francisco. These are reflected in reports of our cohort which indicate that the volume of sexual contacts, as well as the likelihood of behaviors which are thought to transmit disease and the probable AIDS virus, have been on a downward trend, at least since November 1983 and very probably for a longer period. Our findings suggest that, to a great extent, the sexual choices of our cohort are organized by the desire to avert risk. The steepest trends are among high-risk activities: sex with strangers, sex which involves the exchanges of body fluids that may contain infectious agents, and sex in places that promote multiple partner contacts.[47]

At the very least this shows that gay men can and will reduce their high-risk activities. Had they received the necessary information earlier, their high-risk behavior might have changed in concert with that information. It is important to note that to initiate a significant decline in high-risk behavior, one need not actually close the baths. The baths in San Francisco were not closed until October 1984. Yet, there was evidence of significant behavior change as early as November 1983. All that is necessary is to educate. The assumption that drastic paternalistic measures are necessary in order to change behavior is not substantiated by the McKusick study. Such action may reduce high-risk behavior, but perhaps only as an indirect consequence of the high level of exposure to information that such controversial measures precipitate. In fact, an important venue for the dissemination of this information is the baths and the sex clubs.

IV Drug-users

The gay community are politically sophisticated and have been quick, even if at times misguided, in mobilizing resources on their own behalf. When finally informed about the risks connected with certain kinds of sexual activities they have altered their behavior. Disseminating information to gay men is a relatively easy matter mainly because they are a highly political group who have formed a number of community and professional organizations. The same is not true of IV drug-users and this makes it difficult to get information to them. Efforts to inform IV-users about HIV/AIDS and about ways to minimize their risk for it have been slow and not particularly vigorous. This, in part, is due to the fact that IV-users are thought to be uneducable by mainstream society. But recent studies show that this assumption is false. IV-users have become well informed, for the most part, and have made behavioral changes to avoid AIDS.[48]

In a 1985 New Jersey Health Survey, 577 IV-users attending treatment clinics were asked what the source of their information was (multiple answers were permitted). Of those surveyed, 78% reported that they obtained their information from television, 59% from radio and 69% from newspapers. 38% received their information from a pamphlet, 33% from a drug program and 15% from a drug program field worker. These figures show that most IV-users obtain their information not from sources directed specifically at them, treatment clinics, and so on, but from the mainstream media. Responses to a question about how an IV-user can reduce the risk of getting AIDS are also interesting. 82% answered by avoiding sharing a needle, whereas only 29% knew that soaking a needle in a solution of household bleach and water could sterilize it. From the point of view of an IV-user, it is helpful to know that one should not share needles, but not as helpful as knowing that it is possible to easily sterilize injection equipment. Being told not to share needles when the context will permit nothing else is tantamount to being told not to use needles at all. As the researchers of the above study note:

> [T]here has never been a systematic effort to educate drug abusers about the hazards of needle sharing or the means of attempting to keep their drug paraphernalia clean. In the past, there has only been one message - if you use drugs you should enter treatment; if you do not go into treatment, then whatever ill befalls you will be your own fault.[49]

In the late seventies and early eighties neither gay men nor IV-users had the information they needed to make fully informed and autonomous choices about high-risk actions. In part, this is because the information that was needed was just not available. There is, however, also evidence that when the information did become available, public health authorities were not doing all that they could to convey it to those at highest risk for HIV/AIDS. A similar criticism holds with respect to some factions within the gay community.

IV Drug-use, Disadvantaged Minorities and Adaptive Preferences

I have looked at the social conditions that might account for the sharing of injection equipment among IV drug-users. There is some indication that the prohibition on narcotic use has much to do with the practice of needle-sharing. With respect to IV drug-users, it is also important to ask what draws them to narcotics. Why take drugs at all? The answer to this question reveals that again social conditions should be scrutinized carefully.

In the US there is a disproportionate percentage of AIDS cases among Blacks and Hispanics; 26% of the adult cases that have been reported have been among Blacks and 53% of the pediatric cases have been among Black children. This is startling in view of the fact that Blacks constitute only 11.6% of the US population. Hispanics constitute only 6.5% of the US population, but 14% of adult AIDS cases and 23% of pediatric ones.[50] The disproportionate prevalence of AIDS among these two minority groups reflects higher rates of the disease among Black and Hispanic IV-users, their sexual partners and their infants.[51] It would not be surprising if one of the reasons why a disproportionate number of American Blacks and Hispanics are getting AIDS is that a disproportionate number of Blacks and Hispanics are IV drug-users.

If this is so, it is worth asking why so many Blacks and Hispanics are drawn to drugs. Certainly there may be a connection between poverty and drug-use. This connection between narcotics and poverty is eloquently discussed by James McMearn in an essay entitled "Radical and Racial Perspectives on the Heroin Problem":[52]

> The feelings and attitudes that dominate our disadvantaged black communities are the outgrowth of a nation that turned a deaf ear to cries of poverty,

inequality, injustice, alienation, war, racism, and other conditions that are inconsistent with human dignity. My young black brothers and sisters experience these physically and mentally impoverishing conditions in a land where 70 per cent of our national budget goes for defense. These young people find their only relief in heroin. The poorest ghetto dwellers keep themselves narcotized to keep from having to face their miserable existence. Tragically, for too many of these dwellers the relief has become a permanent escape.

Faced with miserable lives and disillusioned about prospects for the future many ghetto Blacks turn to narcotics. The same is no doubt true for American Hispanics. This theme, that narcotic use is a mechanism for coping with frustration and disappointment, is echoed in a book entitled *Self-Attitudes and Deviant Behavior:*

Thus, the drug subculture may provide the person with a set of values more easily approximated than previously held values. As the individual approximates these newly found values his self-acceptance increases.... [T]he person may find insulation against, and social support for the rejection of, the value system of the broader society by the standards of which he failed. By rejecting the standards by which he failed, the subject at the same time rejects the basis for his self-devaluing judgments.[53]

On this analysis individuals who are unable to succeed by the lights of society turn to the drug sub-culture where the criteria for success are more easily achieved. Self-acceptance, or put differently, self-esteem, which only suffers according to the criteria of mainstream society, flourishes according to that of the sub-culture. Another way of analyzing this phenomenon is with the familiar notion of an *adaptive preference*. Blacks, who regard as poor their chances of fulfilling desires which require the cooperation of mainstream society, experience frustration, low self-esteem and unhappiness. Rather than continue to have crucial desires thwarted, they cultivate desires for a life which they have some hope of satisfying. Again, it is important to keep in mind that cultivating alternative desires because one does not have a chance to satisfy other desires, is not autonomous. The adaptive desires, rather than reflecting what the individual *really* wants, are generated by external conditions. A restriction on what desires can be satisfied gives rise to new desires which are more easily satisfied. Discrimination against Blacks and Hispanics, poverty and ghetto life, all conspire to convey the message that certain doors are closed to these people. Similar conditions foster narcotic use elsewhere. In Britain, for example, an increasing percentage of drug addicts are drawn from the lower middle class.[54]

Black and Hispanic IV drug-users endure a twofold infringement on their autonomy. First, their options to enjoy the fruit of the *American way* are reduced and so they turn to one of the few remaining viable options, the drug sub-culture. Second, having cultivated desires which they have some hope of satisfying, desires associated with the drug sub-culture, they are then placed in the position of having to engage in the very hazardous practice of having to share injection equipment.

The Blame the Victim Syndrome

I have shown that the high-risk actions of IV-users and gay men are less than fully autonomous. Thus from the perspective of the *weak harm principle* interference designed to stop the spread of the virus can be justified.

That is, some forms of intervention, which would have been precluded had the high-risk actions of gay men and IV-users turned out to be fully autonomous, might now be justified on the grounds that the risky behavior was not performed autonomously. Perhaps most importantly, I showed that the wider social milieu in which gay men live is one of the factors which leads them to search for alternative ways of conducting their sexual lives. It is not certain that they would not have adopted these same high-risk activities in a society which didn't discriminate, but Bell and Weinberg claimed that personal long-term relationships are crucial for homosexual men and women; they are at least as important as for heterosexual men and women. Certainly, when we look at what features are sought in a bathhouse by gay men, safety and an out of the way location were among the most important considerations listed.

In addition to showing that the high-risk behavior of gay men was not, and to the extent that it still exists,[55] is not performed autonomously, another important point emerges. There is a causal connection between 1) social attitudes and conditions and 2) frequent impersonal sex. Gay men might well have cultivated desires for long-term monogamous intimacies or other less hazardous ways of conducting their sexual lives had they the same opportunities as heterosexuals. There is, however, also a causal connection between 2) frequent impersonal sex and 3) HIV/AIDS. Individuals with many sexual partners are at increased risk for the virus. On the basis of the connection between 2) and 3) many people would conclude that gay men ought to be held responsible for the prevalence of HIV/AIDS in their community. They blame the victim, but they are wrong. People who take the *blame the victim* line fail to see that there is also a causal relationship among 1), 2) and 3). This point needs to be highlighted. Society is arranged in such a way that it fosters a desire for frequent impersonal sex in gay men; this desire, along with the actions that follow it, has in turn put gay men at high risk for HIV/AIDS. Thus society is indirectly responsible for the fact that this devastating disease has struck the gay community. Those who blame the victim might well benefit from looking at the causal role that they have played in this tragedy.

Society could be organized differently. It could be organized so that it fosters monogamous and low-risk relationships among gay men. To do this it would have to encourage homosexual marriage, perhaps by providing tax incentives, and displaying public service announcements which celebrate the virtues of gay marriage. It might also attempt to educate heterosexuals about homosexuality so that they may look upon homosexual displays of affection and love with the same benevolent eye as they do heterosexual ones. If there is a sincere interest in ensuring that gay men can make autonomous choices and are not *forced* into potentially fatal high-risk choices, such measures will have to be considered seriously. Of course, these changes are not imminent, and they certainly aren't going to help those gay men who are now HIV positive, who are in the last stages of AIDS or who have died from the disease.

What about IV drug-users? I have shown that there is a causal connection between 1) social conditions and 2) needle-sharing. Were narcotics readily and legally available to IV drug-users they would not need to share needles.[56] There is, however, also a causal connection between 2) needle-sharing and 3) HIV/AIDS. Just as the *blame the victim* argument is wrongly invoked in the case of gay men, so it is wrongly invoked in the case of IV drug-users. Those who would appeal to it fail to note the connection among 1), 2) and 3). They fail to note how

95

social conditions, such as poverty and racial discrimination, contribute to the formation of the desire that many people have to take drugs in the first place.

NOTES

1. Richard D. Mohr in 'AIDS, Gays and State Coercion', *Bioethics*, (1987), vol. 1, no. 1, pp. 35-50, supports this conclusion with respect to gay men. He does, however, provide different arguments for it.

2. Mohr, in his article 'AIDS, Gays and State Coercion' and later in his book, *Gays/Justice: A Study of Ethics, Society and Law*, Columbia University Press, New York, (forthcoming), speaks of *independent agents* and their right to voluntary associations. He does not define the notion of an *independent agent* and I am not sure how much normative baggage it carries with it. The difference between Mohr's position and mine is that in addition to looking at whether or not an action is performed voluntarily (independently), I look at whether or not it is performed autonomously. The latter is a stronger criterion for evaluating actions than independence. Indeed, the desires which lead to high-risk may be non-autonomous ones - perhaps *adaptive preferences*. This point has significant implications for social policy. If gay men are acting independently, but non-autonomously, for reasons which have to do with how society is arranged, then the burden may fall on society to change the situation.

3. For extensive discussion of the concept of *autonomy* and of the notion of *autonomy* that I use, see the following articles. Robert Young, 'Autonomy and the Inner Self', *American Philosophical Quarterly*, (1980), vol. 17, no. 1; Gerald Dworkin, 'Autonomy and Behavior Control', *Hastings Center Report*, (1976), vol. 6, no. 1; Harry Frankfurt, 'Freedom of Will and Concept of a Person', *Journal of Philosophy*, (1971), vol. 68.

4. Dworkin, 'Autonomy and Behavior Control', p. 25.

5. I do think, however, that heterosexuals have a wider range of sexual lifestyle options from which to choose. Given this, they also have an increased opportunity to make an autonomous choice.

6. Jon Elster in *Sour Grapes: Studies in the Subversion of Rationality*, Cambridge University Press, Cambridge, (1983), discusses at length the implications of this psychological phenomenon for social and political philosophy.

7. This is not to say that someone with an *adaptive preference* can never act autonomously. If an *adaptive desire* is endorsed by the person who has it, then it might well be autonomous. I would add that for an *adaptive preference/desire* to be autonomous not only must the desire itself be endorsed, but it must be endorsed as an *adaptive desire*. That is, individuals must be aware that the desire which they are endorsing is an adaptive one.

8. See for example Joseph Raz, *The Morality of Freedom*, Clarendon Press, Oxford, (1986), Chapter 14.

9. Sandra Bartky, 'On Psychological Oppression', in *Philosophy and Women*, S. Bishop and M. Weinzweig (eds), Wadsworth Publishing Co., Belmont, Calif., (1979), p. 34. I wish to thank Gerald Doppelt for bringing this article to my attention.

10. For a discussion of the importance of the notion of "psychological oppression" for the physician/patient relationship please see Patricia Illingworth, 'The Friendship Model of Physician/Patient Relationship and Patient Autonomy', *Bioethics*, (1988), vol. 2, no. 1, pp. 22-36.

11. It may also be the case, although this is more controversial, that society has a positive duty to enhance people's capacities for autonomy.

12. Joel Feinberg, *Harm to Self*, Oxford University Press, New York, (1986), p. 12.

13. Incompetency, coercion and ignorance are often thought to be standard obstacles to voluntariness (see for example Joel Feinberg, *Harm to Self*, p. 115). I use them here as ways to assess autonomy basically because they direct attention to issues which are relevant to autonomy.

14. These practices are not, of course, exclusive to gay men; nor do all gay men include them in their sexual repertory.

15. My hunch is that this position is motivated by the desire to maintain the *fast track* which many gay men view as essential to gay liberation.

16. Of course, if one's monogamous partner were infected, then the risk of anal sex with a condom might be greater than the risk of anal sex with a variety of partners both infected and uninfected. I wish to thank Margaret Duckett and Norbert Gilmore for this point.

17. William L. Heyward and James W. Curran, 'The Epidemiology of AIDS in the US', *Scientific American*, (October 1988), vol. 259, no. 4, p. 78.

18. The issue of what constitutes a competent decision is a complicated one which has received extensive discussion by people working in medical ethics and the law. Even the minimal condition which I identify here is not perfectly clear-cut. For example, it is not clear which of the many consequences that might follow an action an agent must be able to identify, in order to be said to be competent. These are important foundational issues. However, this is not the place to address them. I wish to thank Jim Hankinson for helpful discussion of this point.

19. See Benjamin Freedman, 'Competence, Marginal and Otherwise: Concepts and Ethics', *International Journal of Law and Psychiatry*, (1981), vol. 4, pp. 53-72.

20. Harry Frankfurt makes some interesting points about the autonomy of addicts in his paper, 'Freedom of Will and Concept of a Person', pp. 5-20.

21. Some gay men who continue to practice unsafe sex claim that they do so because, when they have unsafe sex, they are either intoxicated or under the influence of drugs. It has been suggested to me that under these conditions gay men are not competent to choose unsafe sex. The same arguments that apply to drug-addicts with a desire for a *fix* apply to gay men with a desire for unsafe sex and I would draw the same conclusion about them. I wish to thank Norbert Gilmore for drawing my attention to this point and for a lively discussion of it.

22. This argument does not show that an addict is competent. What it suggests is that a person, when competent, might decide to become an addict. If so, then we may have an obligation to honour that decision. I wish to thank Jim Hankinson for discussion of this point.

23. Although it would be a mistake to assume universal incompetence among high-risk takers, it might still be the case that some individual members of the high-risk groups are indeed incompetent to make high-risk choices.

24. I do not mean to imply that *all* gay men have a desire for frequent impersonal sex. Some gay men have desires for monogamous relationships, and some for semi-monogamous relationships, etc. The crux of the problem is that these options are not as *real* for gay men as they are for heterosexuals.

25. Alan P. Bell and Martin S. Weinberg, *Homosexualities: A Study of Diversity Among Men and Women*, Simon and Schuster, New York, (1978), p. 239.

26. Martin S. Weinberg and Colin J. Williams, 'Gay Bathhouses and the Social Organisation of Impersonal Sex', *Social Problems*, (1975), vol. 23, no. 2, pp. 125-6.

27. John Rechy, *The Sexual Outlaw*, Grove Press, New York, (1977), p.

28. My attention was drawn to this book by Dennis Altman, *AIDS in the Mind of America*, Anchor Press/Doubleday, New York, (1986), p. 143.

28. David Black, *The Plague Years: A Chronicle of AIDS, the Epidemic of our Times*, Simon and Schuster, New York, (1985), p. 137.

29. Weinberg and Williams, 'Gay Bathhouses and the Social Organisation of Impersonal Sex', p. 125.

30. Bell and Weinberg, *Homosexualities: A Study of Diversity Among Men and Women*, p. 102.

31. Don C. Des Jarlais, Samuel R. Friedman and David Strug, 'AIDS and Needle Sharing Within the IV- Drug Use Subculture', in *The Social Dimensions of AIDS Method and Theory*, D. A. Feldman and T. M. Johnson (eds), Praeger, New York, (1986), p. 114.

32. Ibid., pp. 114-15.

33. Although it is not stated explicitly in this passage that the *number 25 needle* is being shared among the men, only one needle is mentioned and it does seem to be central to the success of the event.

34. Ibid., p. 116.

35. Ibid.

36. Ibid., p. 119.

37. I discuss this issue more extensively in Chapter 4, pp. 122-24.

38. *Life*, (July 1985), cover, as cited in Richard D. Mohr, 'AIDS, Gays and State Coercion', *Bioethics*, vol. 1, no. 1, p. 38.

39. Frances Fitzgerald, 'A Reporter at Large - The Castro-II', *New Yorker*, (July (28) 1986), pp. 45-63.

40. Ibid., p. 51.

41. The Castro is an area in San Francisco where a number of gay men live. It is the *home* of San Francisco's gay community.

42. Fitzgerald, 'A Reporter at Large - The Castro II', p. 51.

43. Ibid., p. 52.

44. Ibid., p. 54.

45. Educational formats which use peer pressure or pander to deep-seated fears may also be problematic for autonomy. I discuss this at length in Chapter 5.

46. Emmanuel Dreuilhe, *Mortal Embrace: Living with AIDS*, Linda Coverdale Trans., Hill and Wang, New York, (1988), p. 117.

47. Leon McKusick, J. A. Wiley, T. J. Coates, R. Stall, G. Saika, S. Morin, K. Charles, W. Horstman and M. A. Conant, 'Reported Changes in the Sexual Behavior of Men at Risk for AIDS, San Francisco, 1982-84 - The AIDS Behavioral Research Project', *Public Health Reports*, (November/December 1985), vol. 100, no. 6, p. 628.

48. Samuel R. Friedman, D. C. Des Jarlais and J. L. Sotheran, 'AIDS Health Education for Intravenous Drug Users', *Health Education Quarterly*, (Winter 1986), vol. 13, no. 4, p. 386.

49. Harold M. Ginzburg, J. French, J. Jackson, P. I. Hartsock, M. G. MacDonald and S. H. Weiss, 'Health Education and Knowledge Assessment of HTLV-III Diseases among Intravenous Drug Users', *Health Education Quarterly*, (Winter 1986), vol. 13, no. 4, pp. 379-82.

50. Heyward and Curran, 'The Epidemiology of AIDS in the US', p. 78.

51. Ibid.

52. James H. McMearn, 'Radical and Racial Perspectives on the Heroin Problem' in *"It's So Good, Don't Even Try It Once": Heroin in Perspective*, D. E. Smith and G. R. Gay (eds.), Prentice-Hall, New Jersey, (1972), p. 119.

53. Howard B. Kaplan, *Self-Attitudes and Deviant Behavior*, Goodyear Publishing Company, Pacific Palisades, Calif., (1975), p. 10.

54. John Kaplan, 'Taking Drugs Seriously', *The Public Interest*, (1988), vol. 92, p. 35.

55. Until the social conditions which mandate a sexual life consisting primarily of multiple anonymous sexual encounters change, the context continues to be ripe for *adaptive preference* formation.

56. Some people might want to claim that it isn't necessary to decriminalize narcotic use in order to reduce the spread of the virus among IV drug-users. All one needs to do is provide them with easy access to free sterilized equipment (needle exchange programs). I do not think that this is sufficient. There is some evidence that needle-sharing also functions as a *bonding* mechanism among IV drug-users. There was an element of this in the example I gave of someone *getting his wings*. Such bonding mechanisms may be necessary because narcotic users

constitute a sub-culture. If this is so, then by legalizing narcotics we might reduce not only the drug community's status as a sub-culture, but also the concomitant need for a bonding mechanism.

4

Social Responsibility

Two questions needed to be answered before the moral worthiness of AIDS policies, which would interfere with people's liberty, could be assessed. Those questions were: 1) Are the actions through which HIV/AIDS is transmitted primarily self-regarding or other-regarding? and 2) If the virus is transmitted primarily through self-regarding actions, are those actions performed autonomously?

In Chapter 2, I showed that transmission of HIV/AIDS within the two highest risk groups is primarily a case of self-harm and not harm to others. This is an important point because in the *good society* caution needs to be exercised before interfering with actions that do not have harmful consequences for others. In Chapter 3, the risky behavior of IV drug-users and gay men was seen to be less than fully autonomous. The high-risk choices made by people in these communities were a function *not* of their autonomous desires, but of the reduced options with which they were presented and the psychological mayhem which this reduction in options may have wrought.

The unwary reader may be confused at this point. On the one hand I assert that HIV/AIDS is a self-inflicted harm. Yet, on the other hand, I claim that gay men and IV drug-users do not act autonomously. These two claims are not incompatible. What I have shown is that according to one criterion, HIV/AIDS is a self-inflicted harm, but that according to another crucial criterion for assessing whether or not an action is performed *freely*, it is not a self-inflicted disease. Against the background of this analysis, the more practical matter of AIDS social policy can be addressed.[1]

To justify liberty-limiting social policy in the *good society* either the weak or the strong version of the *harm principle* can be adopted. By showing that transmission of HIV/AIDS within the two highest risk groups is primarily a case of harm to self, I also show that according to the *strong harm principle*, liberty-limiting policies are not justified. Does the *weak harm principle* speak for or against liberty-limiting social policy? In this chapter, I will argue that even on the basis of this stronger criterion for interfering with individual liberty, liberty-limiting policies are not justified. Having established that the high-risk actions of gay men and IV drug-users are not performed autonomously for reasons which have to do with external conditions, namely, social conditions, it is open to advocates of the *weak harm principle* to recommend liberty-limiting social policy. Now the question is, should they avail themselves of this option? The answer to this question is no.

Because those who support the *weak harm principle* are interested in maintaining the autonomy of individuals, they are committed to interfering with liberty *only* when absolutely necessary. I show that according to the long-term goal of this version of the principle, preserving autonomy, it is important to look not just at the fact that some decisions are not autonomous, but also at the specific obstacles to autonomy. In the case at hand, the obstacles to autonomous decision-making are the socially induced desires of gay men and IV drug-users. Given this, and the interest in maintaining autonomy, it would be wrong to adopt AIDS policies which would further interfere with the autonomy of gay men and IV drug-users.

I buttress this position by showing that it is especially important not to saddle those who have already had their autonomy diminished with further diminishments when the original diminishment of autonomy has 1) harmed the individual and 2) been achieved by means which are morally wrong. Before turning to this argument, I want to look at an example of an efficiency-based argument against liberty-limiting policy.

Efficiency-Based Arguments

Many authors have argued against highly intrusive policies such as isolation, quarantine and mandatory testing on the grounds that they would be ineffective.[2] These arguments are founded on cost-benefit analysis. The costs to privacy and liberty are high and the potential for benefit low. Some authors have taken an even stronger stand and argued that some liberty-limiting policies will actually be counter-productive.[3] These arguments are impressive; they successfully show that many policies that are under consideration are not worth the price that society would have to pay for them.

But efficiency-based arguments may not be enough to stop the adoption of liberty-limiting social policy. AIDS has evoked widespread fear, panic and anger. Strong emotions, such as these, may override considerations of efficiency and the importance that has traditionally been attributed to privacy and liberty. Hence, arguments grounded in cost-benefit considerations may not protect persons who have HIV/AIDS from threats to their liberty and autonomy.

Although these arguments are founded on a cost-benefit analysis they remain in the domain of moral arguments. Considerations of liberty and autonomy are weighed along with other considerations. When looking at a particular policy, advocates of efficiency arguments might weigh the benefits of a policy in terms of its capacity to slow the spread of HIV against harms to individual liberty. Consider the following cost-benefit argument against screening.

Screening refers to the practice of mandatory testing for HIV seropositivity of any specific population. A specific population might be everyone in a particular society (universal screening) or everyone in a high-risk target group (selective screening of, say, homosexuals, IV drug-users, prostitutes, prisoners). In their paper, "AIDS Screening, Confidentiality and the Duty to Warn",[4] Larry Gostin and William Curran have argued against screening, in most cases, on efficiency grounds. They endorse the following general criterion for any kind of mandatory selective screening: "selective screening must be based upon the undisputed achievement of the protection of the public health which clearly outweighs the invasion of individual privacy and loss of employment which could result to individuals in these two groups".[5]

To facilitate application of this general principle they introduce a set of criteria which must be satisfied by any proposed program for mandatory screening, if it is to be implemented. These are as follows:

1) The group to be screened must have a reservoir of infection so that there are not disproportionate

numbers of infected persons having to submit to intrusive testing policies.

2) The group to be tested must exist within an environment where there is a significant risk of communicating the virus.

3) The results of the test should be helpful to authorities in reducing the spread of infection and it must be shown that this could not have been achieved without knowledge of the results of testing.

4) The harmful consequences of testing and precautions must not be disproportionate to the benefits.

5) There is no other less intrusive method of achieving the public health goal.[6]

Given this rather rigorous set of criteria there is little chance that the benefit to public health will outweigh the costs associated with screening. Since there is not a treatment or vaccine for the virus it is unlikely that selective screening would satisfy condition 3). That is, it would not slow the spread of the virus. To justify selective screening it would have to be shown that the personal knowledge to be gained from testing will be influential in motivating people to change their behavior. But there is no convincing evidence to support the view that it will do this. Gostin and Curran suggest that screening may have the opposite effect. It may drive those most at risk for HIV away from testing, counselling and treatment[7] because they might well believe, in view of the fact that there is not a cure, that testing may lead to other even more intrusive social policy.

As I argued in Chapter 2, people react differently to different information. Some people who receive bad news about their health may enter into a state of denial and not modify their behavior at all. A few, having received what they view as a *death sentence* may adopt a *what have I got to lose* attitude which, in turn, might lead them to continue unsafe practices. Others may well modify their behavior as a result of discovering their positive antibody status. How particular individuals will react to adverse health information is a matter that depends very much on the particular individual. Mandatory screening, universal or selective, cannot take into account the wide variety of psychological states that characterize individuals. Given this, a policy which risks generating dangerous and adverse reactions, without promising any clear-cut benefits, might well produce more harm than good.

This point is supported by a number of authors. David Mayo has suggested that there could be serious problems because universal mandatory testing would have a large number of false positives and negatives. People with false positives might react in any of the above mentioned ways, some of which would entail that the virus is spread. And persons with false negatives may well infect others because they hold the false belief that they cannot.[8]

The Problem With Efficiency Arguments

Efficiency-based arguments have been advanced against most of the liberty-limiting policies that have been considered: quarantine, isolation, contact-tracing and of course, screening and mandatory testing. Although these arguments are just as strong as the one considered here, they may not be strong enough to quell policies which, though basically inefficient according to the criteria of cost-benefit analysis, are highly invasive of individual liberty.

The problem is that cost-benefit considerations like those used by Gostin and Curran, are not the only ones invoked by policy-makers. It is not uncommon for policy-makers to also take into account political, religious and social considerations. AIDS, if anything, is likely to reinforce this practice. Fear and panic about it have created an atmosphere which is ripe for invasive policies. This atmosphere may have contributed to the fact that policies which do not fare well on the cost-benefit scale are nonetheless under consideration or have already been adopted.

Efficiency-based arguments weigh the costs of adopting a particular policy against the benefit of doing so. When, in a particular case, the costs outweigh the benefits, whatever is at issue is doomed to be either imprudent or not worth the price that would have to be paid for it. In Gostin and Curran's argument costs and benefits were basically of two kinds. The costs were concerned for the most part with privacy and liberty, and the benefits were focused mainly on whether or not screening would be effective in slowing the spread of the virus. As the argument stood, screening was not favored. But there is nothing which prevents the scales from being tipped in the other direction.

New facts about the virus, for example, might tip the cost-benefit scales in favor of liberty-limiting policies. To some, quarantine might be justified if it were discovered that people who are HIV positive are infectious for an identifiable length of time. If a treatment for AIDS were discovered, screening, mandatory testing and contact-tracing might be viewed as more feasible to some than they would be if there were no treatment. Needless to say, more people would willingly embrace the opportunity to be tested were there an effective treatment or vaccine. Coercive measures would not be necessary.

Many people who are concerned about the spread of HIV/AIDS might agree with these policy recommendations and would have no qualms about importing these sorts of considerations into the cost-benefit analysis. But many would not be as comfortable were we to import into the calculus, considerations about allaying fear and anxiety in the general population or satisfying people's primitive desires to retaliate against those who have HIV/AIDS. The point is that there is nothing in cost-benefit arguments restricting what can count as a cost or benefit.

We are surrounded by fear and panic about AIDS. In a recent column in Toronto's *Globe and Mail* Dr Gifford-Jones described some mail that he had received in response to a column he had written on the treatment of AIDS patients in hospitals. In a paraphrase of these letters he has the following to say:

> Ninety-five per cent of replies from the laity condemned the timid approach to the management of the AIDS crisis. Letter after letter stressed that the primary concern should be the human rights of the healthy. They argued it is ludicrous that those with the AIDS virus should have the freedom to remain anonymous and also the freedom to infect others.[9]

Even granting that we don't know how many letters he received and that the people who wrote were responding to a column calling for more stringent policies, these claims are startling. Why didn't more people write in objection to his views?

A recent study done in Canada at the University of Lethbridge reported similarly discouraging results. Only 4% of those surveyed sympathized with persons with AIDS. Many people identified punishment by God and immoral living as the main cause of the disease. Thirty-two per cent of respondents thought that promiscuity and homosexual lifestyle (immoral living) were the root cause of the disease while another 14% suggested that divine retribution was the source of the disease. A few respondents suggested that persons with AIDS be sent to a colony to die. And 26% of those surveyed felt that a child with the disease should not be permitted to go to school.[10]

Equally disturbing views are held by large numbers of Americans. A comprehensive study which canvassed public attitudes in the US to HIV/AIDS was conducted by Robert Blendon and Karen Donelan between 1983 and 1988. They report that "[m]ost Americans see the control of AIDS as requiring some loss of individual privacy and possible restriction on civil rights," and that "[a] substantial minority of Americans see AIDS as a deserved punishment for offensive or immoral behavior and show signs of intolerance and outright hostility to those with the disease."[11] Furthermore, "a substantial minority believe that those with AIDS should not be allowed to live in their neighborhood or community, and they favor landlords having the right to evict those with the disease".[12]

A more vivid depiction of the fear and hysteria that AIDS has wrought was the sight, at the Third International Conference on AIDS, of Washington police wearing bright yellow rubber gloves, as they rounded up demonstrators outside the conference. The public can hardly be expected to understand this disease or to be compassionate towards those who have it when the police in America's capital show little sign of these virtues. Nor did this incident go unobserved by those who have AIDS. Emmanuel Dreuilhe certainly noticed it:

> When the police in the nation's capital put on plastic gloves before arresting lesbian demonstrators, can I be wrong in thinking that for much of the population we have become beings as frightening as zombies in a horror film, creatures that many wouldn't hesitate to strike down, as in the *Night of the Living Dead*, having once persuaded themselves that we were monsters with empty eyes, despite our

human appearance, and intent on dragging them down with us into the abyss?[13]

It is also worth recalling that as Elizabeth Taylor addressed the National Press Club in Washington a gate crasher held up a sign which read "Quarantine Manhattan Island, the AIDS Capital of the World".

There are more sobering incidents that bear witness to the fear that envelops society. The Rays, a Florida family, had their home destroyed by a fire because their three sons were hemophiliacs known to have been in contact with the virus. Their sons had also been barred from school. Mrs Mowery, a Tennessee woman appearing before a Presidential Commission on HIV/AIDS described the following scenario about her son:

Dwayne has hemophilia and is also learning-disabled... He is HIV positive and was exposed to the virus through contaminated blood products he takes to control his blood clotting. He does not have AIDS now.... The school board did not want my child in school. The most vocal opponent on the board has been a doctor who should know better.[14]

Mrs Mowery tried to sneak her son into school, but gave up after a few days because as she says "When people drive past your house with signs saying 'Kill him, Kill him, Kill him', you have to be afraid."[15]

Nor should the evidence of personal experience be ignored. Many of us have known or heard stories about people being evicted from their homes or fired from their jobs. These examples show that fear of HIV/AIDS, and the attending panic, continue to be widespread. The real problem is that fear, panic and anger may lead people to underestimate the value of liberty and respect for others and to adopt policies which they find more comforting and likely to dispel their fears, policies which, in more reflective moments, they might reject. But more to the point, there is nothing in the efficiency-based arguments which prohibits importing these sorts of considerations into the calculation. If they are imported into it they may well tip the scales against the liberty of gay men and IV drug-users.

Beyond Efficiency: Autonomy, Self-Esteem and Equal Opportunity in the Good Society

The high-risk behavior of gay men and IV drug-users can plausibly be explained by looking at social conditions. Because of certain conditions the behavior which has placed members of these two communities at risk for HIV/AIDS could not be taken to be entirely autonomous.

Questions about autonomy are important, from the point of view of the *weak harm principle*, because they tell us when interference with someone's self-regarding actions is permissible and when it is not. According to the *weak harm principle*, our duty not to interfere with self-regarding behavior holds only with respect to fully autonomous actions. That is, actions which are not autonomous can be interfered with. For example, it might be argued by those who endorse the *weak harm principle* that bathhouses ought to be closed given that attendance at them is not autonomous. In the following, I will argue that although there is good reason to think that the high-risk behavior of gay men and IV-users is not performed autonomously, even from the point of view of the *weak harm principle*, interference with it is not justified.

The Weak Harm Principle and Individual Autonomy

Those who subscribe to the *weak harm principle* want to be sure that decisions and actions are performed autonomously. If a certain action does not meet this condition then interference is justified just so that autonomy is reinstated. There are problems with this position.

For one thing, individuals can benefit in important ways from their non-autonomous choices. The capacity to be autonomous is a skill that can be honed only with practice and experience. A policy which forces people to be autonomous by respecting only their autonomous desires denies them crucial opportunities to refine their autonomy skills through the experience of coming to be autonomous on their own.[16] The *weak harm principle*, by respecting only autonomous decisions, does not give people the opportunity to cultivate their capacity to be autonomous. Taken to an extreme it may destroy the conditions necessary to attain the goal it is designed to realize.

This point needs to be underscored. Imagine that it were possible to accurately determine whether or not a decision is autonomous and that only autonomous decisions were respected. In other words, people would only be allowed to act in ways which were harmful to themselves if they autonomously chose to do so. It goes without saying that people would be prevented from doing a wide variety of things which they now do. For example, Bob would not be allowed to smoke; Joan would not be permitted to eat that extra piece of chocolate mousse cake and Mrs Robinson could not have that affair with Benjamin. The list goes on. There are many reasons why such a scenario is disturbing which I shall not discuss. From the point of view of autonomy, it is especially problematic. If people are denied opportunities to act in non-autonomous ways they are, to all intents and purposes, denied an opportunity to be autonomous. Without opportunities to experiment with different options (smoking, overeating, infidelity) they cannot come to know what options are suited to them. Sometimes, personal experience is the best way to discover whether or not one endorses a particular desire.

Second, respect for persons requires that the whole person be respected and not just that part of the person which is autonomous; it requires that a person be given the freedom to make choices which he might later disavow and also to develop his own autonomy in a way which is authentic to him.

The main problem with this version of the *harm principle* is that by respecting only autonomous desires, it denies important aspects of the person. By taking as crucial whether or not a desire is autonomous, it undermines the very capacity that allows people to come to have autonomous desires. If the *weak harm principle* were the rule rather than the exception, there would be few autonomous desires to respect because the capacity to be autonomous would not develop to an extent sufficient to allow individuals to cultivate these desires.

But even if one endorses the *weak harm principle* it does not follow that interference with the liberty of gay men and IV-users is justified. This point needs to be highlighted. Although the relevant behavior is primarily self-regarding (no one is harmed unless he chooses to be harmed) and the behavior which is causally linked to the harm (HIV/AIDS) is not performed autonomously, it does not follow that the liberty of gay men and IV-users ought to be interfered with. Those who support the *weak harm principle* argue that in the *good society* there is a duty to respect only the autonomous (and self-regarding) choices that people make because they are interested in maintaining and enhancing the individual autonomy.[17] The conclusion that AIDS liberty-limiting policies are justified according to the *weak harm principle* fails to take into account one very important consideration. Namely, that the autonomy of gay men and IV drug-users has been diminished by factors which have much more to do with social conditions than with individual gay men and IV drug-users. If I am right about this, then autonomous decision-making can be reinstated by changing the relevant social conditions. If this option is available, then according to the value the *weak harm principle* itself places on autonomy, it would be morally wrong not to take it. Hence, even from the point of view of this version of the *harm principle* it is wrong to interfere with liberty when autonomy can be reinstated through means which do not interfere with it.

Socially Induced Desires and Social Responsibility

There are other reasons why it would be wrong to interfere with the liberty of gay men and IV drug-users with AIDS liberty-limiting policy. First, members of these two communities have already endured more than enough harm because of social conditions. Second, even if it is granted that some harm to individuals is inevitable in the *good society*, that harm should not occur through mechanisms which are morally reprehensible.

The harm to gay men and IV drug-users has come about through adaptive preferences. By narrowing the options open to gay men and IV drug-users society has induced certain desires in them. Obviously this kind of thing happens all the time. Many of the consumer desires that people have are a function of prevailing social conditions.

For example, a yuppie's desire for a BMW is probably due, in large part, to how society is arranged. But no one concludes that society has wronged the yuppie or that it has a moral duty to extend special consideration to the yuppie's plight. Why should the socially induced desires of gay men and IV drug-users be treated any differently than the socially induced desires of the yuppie?

The yuppie's BMW-desire and the gay man's desire for a freewheeling sexual life are alike in that both are fostered by social conditions and unalike in that our intuitions about what society owes to each differ. It is at least plausible in the case of gay men and IV drug-users that society is morally culpable for the diminishment of autonomy whereas it is counter-intuitive to think that this is so in the case of the yuppie-desire. By comparing these two cases, we can see what, specifically, it is about the socially induced desires of gay men and IV drug-users that indicate that society is morally responsible for the creation of their desires.[18]

Harm and Socially Induced Desires

The most obvious difference between the socially induced desire for a freewheeling sexual life and the socially induced desire for a BMW is that the former, unlike the latter, is extremely harmful to the person who has it. A worst case scenario for the yuppie is that he or she suffer from the extreme stress associated with doing what has to be done in order to be in the financial position to buy the BMW. In some rare instances, this might mean enduring a heart attack. The consequences for a gay man of his socially induced desire for the *fast track* have included HIV infection and AIDS. This means that for all too many gay men a consequence of their socially induced desire for a certain kind of sexual lifestyle is death. Certainly, one of the reasons for thinking that society is culpable for its role in creating the desire for a free-wheeling sexual lifestyle is the severity of the harm to gay men of that desire.

A similar line of reasoning holds for IV drug-users. Not only is there a correlation between narcotic use and minority status, but in addition, a correlation between prohibiting narcotics, sharing needles and coming into contact with HIV/AIDS. This suggests that social conditions are responsible for the desire to take drugs as well as the desire to share needles. Moreover, the harm to IV drug-users is compounded by the prohibitions on narcotic use mainly because drug laws make it impossible to exercise any quality control on illegal substances.

> Consumers of heroin and the various synthetic substances sold on the street face ... severe consequences, including fatal overdoses and poisonings from unexpectedly potent or impure drug supplies. More often than not, the quality of a drug addict's life depends greatly upon his or her access to reliable supplies. Drug-enforcement operations that succeed in temporarily disrupting supply networks are thus a double-edged sword: they encourage some addicts to seek admission into drug-treatment programs, but they oblige others to seek out new and hence less reliable suppliers; the result is that more, not fewer, drug-related emergencies and deaths occur.[19]

Thus drug-addicts experience a twofold harm. Social conditions contribute to the formation of the desire to take drugs. Then laws which prohibit narcotic use make the practice of taking illicit drugs extremely hazardous because of needle-sharing and the absence of quality control.

The crux of the harm argument has little to do with the fact that the harmed groups are also highly stigmatized.

Our moral intuitions would be the same if it were the case that as a result of a socially induced desire yuppies suffered severe harm. Imagine the following. Suppose that the socially induced desire to drive a BMW turned out to be extremely risky. Imagine that 1 out of every 100 times a yuppie slipped the key into the ignition, the beautiful BMW, including the yuppie, blew up. Would we not, given this scenario, hold the source of this desire morally responsible for cultivating it?

This comparison shows that, of the desires that are socially induced, there is an inclination to hold society morally responsible for those that saddle individuals with harm. When there is no severe harm to the individual as a result of holding the desire, there is no compelling reason to hold society responsible. In the case of the high-risk choices made by gay men and IV-users the harm is serious enough to commend social culpability.

Not only are gay men and IV drug-users harmed by their *adaptive desires*, but they have very little to gain from having these desires. This too distinguishes them from the yuppie. Consider the benefits of having the desires for those who are saddled with them. In some cases society confers sufficient benefits on those who assume the desires to justify the risks associated with them. This is probably the case with the yuppie's desire for a BMW. Although there are the harms associated with yuppie-stress, which come about from having the desire, there are also social rewards to be had. In return for the yuppie's cultivation of the BMW-desire, he gains social acceptance, respect and high self-esteem (not to mention a shiny, new BMW). The same is not true for the gay man who cultivates the socially induced desire for the *fast track* or ghetto Blacks who come to desire narcotics. Not only are they not showered with respect and admiration for cultivating the desires and requisite behavior, but they are often blamed

119

for having them. Princess Anne, proponent of the *blame the victim* position, bears witness to this in her comments about AIDS. The following is a precis of Princess Anne's view.

> [W]hy on earth should homosexuals (the main carriers, whose sexual practices and promiscuity are tailor-made for transmitting the disease) regard themselves, or be regarded by others, as victims? We do not talk of *syphilis victims* or *herpes victims*, or *gonorrhoea victims*. We regard the majority of those who contract these diseases as suffering the consequences of their own voluntary acts. It is surely the same with AIDS.[20]

Princess Anne is not unique in believing that gay men are to be blamed for their promiscuous lifestyle and, in turn, for AIDS. She ignores the role that society has played in creating the crucial desires. Unlike the yuppie, the gay man is condemned by society for the very desires which society has fostered. Unlike the yuppie, he is not rewarded for his cooperation, but punished. Finally, unlike the yuppie, he has very little to gain from society for coming to have the socially induced desire.

Socially Induced Desires and Morally Problematic Means
There is another reason why society should be held morally responsible for the socially induced desires of gay men and IV-users and for the subsequent harm that befell them. If, in fostering a desire, society violates certain moral principles which are taken to be fundamental, then not only has it fostered the desire, but it has done so wrongfully. Suppose that the mechanism society uses to induce a desire were morally neutral or even morally praiseworthy. For example, one way to induce people to adopt healthy habits is to inform them of the pleasures which attend a more virtuous life. This would be much

less problematic than the opposite scenario, one in which the means used to induce the desire violated some fundamental moral principle.[21]

Equal Opportunity

Discriminatory laws, regulations and intolerance toward homosexuals deny them an equal opportunity to express their sexuality and intimacy preferences. Monogamous relationships, either long-term or sequential, are not as viable an option for gay men as they are for heterosexuals. This is so, in part, because society does not encourage and promote (let alone tolerate) romantic liaisons among homosexuals in the same way as it does heterosexuals. Same sex relationships are not sanctioned by society through tax benefits, joint health insurance policies or other state plans which reward heterosexuals. In some places sodomy continues to be against the law. Effectively, what society has done is to put severe obstacles in the way of gay men choosing a life-plan that suits them.

Promoting some conceptions of the *good life* over others has the consequence of favoring some life-plans over others. To the extent that some life-plans are given a preferred status over others, those that are not preferred lose their status as real alternatives. This, in turn, discourages people from making decisions for conceptions which are not favored. Discrimination against same sex predispositions is a good example of this.

The only *real* sexual lifestyle option open to gay men is the one many of them have chosen, multiple anonymous sexual encounters. This is not to say that it is impossible for a gay man to choose an alternative sexual lifestyle, but to say that it is more difficult for him to do so. Nor does the position I support condemn frequent anonymous sex as an option. My view is not that no one ought to choose multiple anonymous sex as a way of conducting their sexual lives, but that no one ought to be *forced* to choose it, for lack of other viable options. As things stand now, gay men have very few sexual lifestyle options from which to choose. This makes remote the possibility of choosing autonomously the *fast track* or any other sexual lifestyle; the circumstances are ripe for adaptive preference formation.

That people are given equal opportunities to develop their particular conceptions of the *good life* is important for a number of reasons. In the *good society*, the state is designed to foster social conditions which will allow individuals to pursue their own life-plans and conceptions of the *good life*.[22] Fairness considerations require that all life-plans have an equal standing with respect to the state (that is, that the state not favor some over others) at least in so far as they do not harm others. Doing otherwise violates the basic tenet of neutrality among conceptions of the *good*, and in turn, denies everyone within a particular society the benefits of pluralism.

Paternalistic Legislation

Laws which prohibit the private use of narcotics are paternalistic. In a society committed to respecting individual autonomy they constitute a harm on this ground alone because violations to autonomy are in and of themselves harms. In view of much of the crime and corruption alleged to be associated with narcotics, the idea that drug-use is a self-regarding action may strike some as surprising. How can anything which appears to have such obviously harmful consequences for society be construed as a self-regarding activity?

It is important to distinguish the harms connected with drug-use from those connected with prohibitions on it. In the US, laws which prohibit the private consumption of narcotics are costly and, as Ethan Nadelmann has argued, counter-productive.[23] The crime and corruption associated with drugs are more a function of the laws against drugs than of the drugs themselves. Consider the following. If drug laws were repealed, the producing, selling, buying and consuming of narcotics would no longer be criminal activities. Similarly, the crimes drug-users commit in order to obtain the money to purchase expensive illicit drugs would decrease dramatically. If drugs were legal substances, as alcohol is, they would become much less expensive and the crimes which are now executed in order to purchase them would become unnecessary.[24]

Drug-related violence in the form of violent crimes committed by people under the influence of narcotics is another kind of criminal activity associated with drugs. Some drugs may have the effect of increasing violent behavior. But Nadelmann points out that it is just not clear yet whether or not drugs such as *crack* contribute to an increase in violent behavior. He also very astutely points out that "no illicit drug is as widely associated with violent behavior as alcohol."[25] It may also be the case that the violent behavior which is thought to be fostered by drugs would diminish with the decriminalization and regulation of drugs. If drugs were regulated in the same way that alcohol is, some quality control could be exercised. The violence associated with drugs might diminish as the quality was enhanced.

Many of the harmful consequences which illicit drug-use is thought to be responsible for would more accurately be attributed to drug laws and the *war* on drugs. If this is so, then drug-use should remain in the self-regarding camp and laws which prohibit it should be rightly described as paternalistic interferences. According to the *strong harm principle* such interference is wrong because it fails to respect the individual claims of people to do what they want in areas which concern only themselves.

Laws prohibiting narcotic use do not fare much better with the *weak harm principle*. Although the primarily self-regarding activity of taking illicit drugs may not be performed autonomously, this diminishment in autonomy can in many cases accurately be ascribed to external social conditions such as poverty, racism and a lack of opportunities for social mobility. So even on the *weak harm principle* paternalistic laws which prohibit drug-use constitute wrongful interference in people's lives.

Self-Esteem and the Good Society

To successfully pursue one's conception of the *good life*, an individual must have self-esteem.[26] Self-esteem is composed of a combination of internal and external factors. John Rawls provides the following description of self-respect/self-esteem:

> First of all ... it [self-respect] includes a person's sense of his own value, his secure conviction that his conception of his good, his plan of life, is worth carrying out. And second, self-respect implies a confidence in one's ability, so far as it is within one's power, to fulfill one's intentions. When we feel that our plans are of little value, we cannot pursue them with pleasure or take delight in their execution. Nor plagued by failure and self-doubt can we continue in our endeavors.[27]

Self-esteem and self-respect have to do, at least in part, with how one's life-plans and capacities to engage in them are viewed by others. This suggests that how society views different conceptions of the *good* will affect the level of

124

self-esteem that individuals can attain. Put differently society is a venue through which self-esteem can be nurtured and enhanced, or discouraged and eliminated. This is not surprising. Most of us are aware, from personal experience, that our self-esteem can be dramatically diminished when, in the eyes of others, our projects are seen as not worth pursuing and our capacities undervalued. Low self-esteem, then, is to some extent within the control of society.[28]

Self-esteem is important because it is essential for achieving the things in life which are generally valued: mutually loving relationships and creative and rewarding work. To have self-esteem people need to believe that the life-plans which they choose are worth pursuing. Society is important here because it determines, to a large extent, whether or not the life-plans with which individuals come to identify are seen as worthwhile. When they are not viewed as worthwhile by society, self-esteem suffers.

Self-esteem, Gay Men and IV Drug-users

Society has made it perfectly clear that from its point of view homosexuality is not to be tolerated and is certainly not something about which to be proud. It has succeeded in conveying the message that homosexuality is something about which one ought to be ashamed. Given social attitudes towards homosexuality one certain way to maintain whatever self-esteem that one has is to prevent information about one's sexual tastes from becoming public. For gay men public knowledge about their sexual preferences often entails more than public contempt; it also entails self-contempt. IV drug-users are viewed with similar disdain; they are often thought to be worthless people who are only a burden on society. In his personal testimony Dreuilhe explains how society's view of both gay men and IV drug-users affects them and their fight against AIDS.

How can homosexuals and drug addicts feel patriotically inspired in their private war when they don't even like themselves, or may actually hate themselves because of a self-image that reflects society's contempt for them? If the opinion of others finally convinces you that you are morally or physically deficient, how can you believe in yourself or in the importance of your own survival? The first reflex of groups stigmatized by society, such as the Jews, is to feel beaten - almost guilty - right from the start, and so they climb meekly into the Nazi's box cars. In the same way, many AIDS patients give up without a fight, as if they felt they were somehow getting only what they deserved.[29]

Dreuilhe's comments stand as a personal confirmation of the view, held by Rawls and others, that society can strongly influence individual self-esteem.

If homosexuality and IV drug-use carry with them a loss of self-esteem, and self-esteem is essential for successfully pursuing one's life-plan, then it is also the case that gay men and IV drug-users do not have an equal opportunity to cultivate their conceptions of the *good life*. If the *good society* has a mandate to be neutral with respect to life-plans, then by denying gay men and IV drug-users access to self-esteem, they have thereby wronged them. Gay men have not had an equal opportunity to cultivate and develop different kinds of relationships, nor, in turn, the capacities that they would need in order successfully to negotiate such relationships. Because their sexuality is viewed with contempt and disdain, they have often not had an opportunity to develop the self-esteem needed to pursue and enjoy different kinds of personal relationships were they to become available.

The self-esteem of IV drug-users is often similarly diminished. In some cases this is because narcotic users, as such, are seen as worthless; in other cases it is because they are often drawn from minority communities that are thought to be worthless; and in still other cases it is simply because IV drug-users are often from working class and poor environments which are viewed as worthless.

Objections and Replies

At this point one might object to the line of reasoning that I have been advancing on the following grounds. One might agree that it is wrong to deny gay men an equal opportunity to realize their life-plans, but argue that it is nonetheless a wrong about which nothing can be done. Hatred of homosexuals is not something that as a society we can change; these attitudes are natural and cannot be changed, and even if they could be, the means needed to make the change is not within the sphere of government. The process of change would itself require more interference with liberty than the liberty it would preserve.

A second objection might go as follows. It might be argued that it most certainly is the case that fear and hatred towards homosexuals can be changed, and that, in fact, it already has changed. Thus, the objection grants that there once was severe discrimination and homophobia, but denies that it still exists. If this is so, then although it may be the case that society once harmed gay men, it is no longer the case.[30] But what follows from this? For this objection to be a significant one with respect to the AIDS crisis, it would also need to be the case that serious discrimination against gay men had ended long before AIDS struck the gay community.

First, it is not at all clear that, even in these more permissive times, discrimination against homosexuals has ended. In a recent study done for the US Department of Justice it was pointed out by Peter Finn and Taylor McNeil that "Homosexuals are the most frequent victims of hate motivated violence, including verbal intimidation, assault and vandalism."[31] In Britain, the *Sunday Telegraph* reported the results of a Gallup Poll which showed that 62% of those polled thought that homosexuality was wrong and 60% that homosexuality should not be an accepted alternative lifestyle.[32]

Also in Britain, the controversial Clause 28 was recently (February 1988) approved by 202 votes to 122, a government majority of 80. It prohibits state schools from promoting "the acceptability of homosexuality as a pretended family relationship".[33] On one interpretation of this Clause local schools would not be permitted to generate an awareness of different sexual orientations.[34] Clause 28 states, in no uncertain terms, that homosexuality is not a legitimate alternative to heterosexuality.

It ensures that homosexuality will not be viewed, within mainstream society, as having equal status with heterosexuality. This is important because it shows that in Britain 1) there is a clear move in the direction of increased discrimination and 2) that the value of neutrality among conceptions of the *good life* is not being respected. The following passage taken from a *Times* commentary on the Clause supports this interpretation.

Society depends on the institution of the family for the care of both children and the elderly and the maintenance of values. It cannot let that institution be relativized away as one of a number of optional lifestyles. At the same time, it has to recognize that the homosexual minority will not go away, and come to terms with it. They (society) can also discriminate

between tolerating individual homosexuals and
surrendering their own value system.[35]
I leave it to others to quibble with the author of this
passage, Digby Anderson. I quote him to provide further
evidence that homosexuality is not viewed as an equal life
option and that homosexuals still suffer from
discrimination. It is also important to note that this
discrimination not only exists as an attitude towards gay
persons, but that it is entrenched in the law. Clause 28
bears witness to this; discrimination against homosexuals
not only exists, but is buttressed by very recent legislation.

Discriminatory legislation is not restricted to Britain. In
the summer of 1986 the US Supreme Court held in *Bowers*
v. *Hardwick* that the American Constitution does not
confer a fundamental right on homosexuals to engage in
sodomy.[36] This means that individual states have the legal
right to prohibit sodomy even between consenting adults.
Michael J. Bowers, the Attorney General for Georgia and
the Petitioner in the case of *Bowers* v. *Hardwick* defends
this decision for reasons which are similar to those given
by Anderson in support of Clause 28. According to
Bowers:

> [H]omosexual sodomy is the anathema of the basic
> units of our society - marriage and the family. To
> decriminalize or artificially withdraw the public's
> expression of its disdain for this conduct does not
> uplift sodomy, but rather demotes these sacred
> institutions to merely other alternative life-styles.[37]

This legislative evidence also speaks to the first objection
that I raised, namely, that discrimination against
homosexuals is something that society cannot change.
Because discrimination against homosexuality is embraced
by the law, it is difficult to take this objection very
seriously. It is one thing to say that the deeply ingrained
hostility to homosexuality cannot be erased, and quite

another to assert this when these attitudes are entrenched in the law. One cannot help but wonder whether or not those who advance the *nothing can be done* argument have a sincere interest in seeing discrimination against homosexuals end. At the very least, it ought to be demanded of someone who claims to object to discrimination against homosexuals that he be prepared to eliminate discriminatory laws.

Discrimination against homosexuals continues to be widespread.[38] Even if this discrimination had ended prior to the advent of AIDS it would not have ended soon enough to have diminished its harmful effects on gay men. In the last chapter I suggested that the high-risk lifestyle embraced by many gay men was a reaction to an extremely oppressive society; it was a movement of liberation. If I am right about this, then even if discrimination had ended altogether prior to AIDS, its detrimental effects were still being experienced by gay men.

AIDS will only make the problem of discrimination against homosexuals worse. In a study done in Scotland on the effects of government AIDS awareness programs there was strong evidence that the public's attitudes towards the two high-risk groups was extremely hostile and that this had been extended to how persons with AIDS are viewed. Hastings, Leather and Scott report the following results.

> [T]he connection between AIDS and homosexuals and drug addicts dominated people's perceptions and largely determined their feelings about the condition.... Both homosexuals and drug addicts were seen as degenerate, strange, and difficult to comprehend. Homosexuals were particularly disliked, with respondents refusing to tolerate behavior which they described as *dirty* and *unnatural*.... These negative feelings were

transferred to AIDS, which was seen as a degenerate, shameful, and almost taboo condition.[39]
The negative attitude held by the general public towards homosexuals and IV drug-users is transferred to persons with AIDS. It would not be at all surprising if in addition to this, the fear and panic associated with AIDS fuels further hostility towards members of both communities.

It would be a mistake to conclude from this that negative attitudes towards persons with AIDS are restricted to the general public or to those who are uneducated about the disease. In this case prejudice is not just a matter of ignorance. A recent study looked at the attitudes of medical students to homosexuals and persons with AIDS.[40] The students were presented with one of four patient scenarios which differed only in how the patient was identified. In two of the scenarios the patient was identified as having either AIDS or leukaemia and in the other two as either homosexual or heterosexual.

The students were then asked to answer a survey which was designed to assess their attitudes to the patients described in the scenario. Students were asked questions of the following sort. 1) Would they be willing to attend a party where the patient prepared the food? 2) Would they be willing to work in the same office as the patient? 3) Would they be willing to have a conversation with the patient? 4) Would they be willing to allow one of their children to visit the patient? The following results were reported. The students were asked to rate their willingness on a scale of 1 to 6 with 1 representing the least favorable and 6 the most. In response to 1) when the patient was identified as an AIDS carrier the mean score among respondents was 4.84, contrasted with a score of 5.55 when the patient was described as having leukaemia. Similarly, when the patient was described as a homosexual leukaemia patient the respondent mean score was 4.88 compared to

5.51 when the patient was described as heterosexual. A similar trend was witnessed with question number 3); respondents tended to have less favorable attitudes to the persons with AIDS and the homosexuals. An even stronger bias against these two groups was witnessed in response to questions 2) and 4). With respect to the former, scores of 4.88/6.00 were reported for the AIDS/leukaemia patients and 5.06 and 5.81 for the homosexual/heterosexual leukaemia patient. And with the latter, respondents scored a 3.31/5.53 for the AIDS/leukaemia patients and a 3.83 and a 5.00 for the homosexual/heterosexual patients.[41] The authors have the following to say about the results of the survey:

> [O]n seven of the 12 prejudice items, the AIDS patients were evaluated much more harshly than the leukemia victims. A similar pattern emerged with respect to sexual preference. Regardless of which disease was involved, the homosexual patients were viewed as being more responsible for their illness ... more dangerous to others ... and suffering less pain than the heterosexual patients....[42]

What this study shows is that discriminatory attitudes against gays and persons with AIDS are not restricted to the ignorant, but extend also to health professionals, those who are well informed about the disease.

The point that I have been making in this chapter and in the last is that a serious wrong has been committed against both gay men and IV drug-users and that as a consequence of this they have suffered. Not only have they endured a serious loss of self-esteem, dignity and liberty, but more recently many of them have developed either a positive HIV status or full-blown AIDS. Many have died from the disease and many more will in the future. This, of course, is terrible for any individual to have to endure. But in the particular case of AIDS the people who have been most affected by the disease are gay men and IV drug-users, individuals who have already suffered enormously and who have been stigmatized by society. For the most part, society has responded to the AIDS crisis and to those who have been struck by it with fear, hatred and hostility. This may explain the reluctance of many governments to fund AIDS research and care for AIDS patients.

The one point that should emerge from the arguments that I have presented is that in view of the harm that society has already inflicted on gay men and IV drug-users further harms are absolutely unjustified from the point of view of the *good society*. Policies, such as contact-tracing, mandatory testing and isolation, infringe on liberty and hence on autonomy. They constitute harms for this reason alone. In the *good society* an individual whose autonomy is not respected is harmed.

The considerations that I have outlined suggest that not only should any social policy which is adopted not further harm gay men and IV drug-users, but should to some extent alleviate some of the harm that they have already experienced. AIDS social policy provides society with a good opportunity to mend some of the suffering that past policies have caused both gay men and IV drug-users. AIDS social policy should not just stop the spread of the virus, but also right some of the wrongs which have been inflicted on gay men and IV drug-users. At the very least what I have shown is that on the two versions of the *harm principle*, such policies are not justified.

NOTES

1. I wish to thank Jim Hankinson for suggesting that I clarify this point.

2. See for example, Margaret Somerville and Norbert Gilmore, *Human Immunodeficiency Virus Antibody Testing*, a publication of the McGill Centre for Medicine, Ethics and Law, (1988); Ruth Macklin, 'Predicting Dangerousness and the Public Health Response to AIDS', *Hastings Center Report*, (1986), vol. 16, no. 6, pp. 16-23.

3. David J. Mayo, 'AIDS Quarantines and Non-compliant Positives': in *AIDS: Ethics and Public Policy*, C. Pierce and D. VanDeVeer (eds), Wadsworth Publishing Co., Belmont, Calif., (1988), pp. 113-23.

4. Larry Gostin and William J. Curran, 'AIDS Screening, Confidentiality, and the Duty to Warn', *American Journal of Public Health*, (March 1987), vol. 77, no. 3, p. 362.

5. Ibid.

6. Ibid.

7. Ibid.

8. Mayo, 'AIDS Quarantines and Non-compliant Positives', p. 117.

9. W. Gifford-Jones, 'Mail on AIDS Victims Shows Strongest Response is Fear', *Globe and Mail*, Toronto, (October (27) 1987).

10. Elaine O'Farrell, 'Canadians Still Harbor Myths and Many Fears about AIDS', *Medical Post*, (September (8) 1987), p. 50.

11. Robert J. Blendon and Karen Donelan, 'Discrimination Against People with AIDS', *New England Journal of Medicine*, (October (13) 1988), vol. 319, no. 15, p. 1023.

12. Ibid., p. 1024.

13. Emmanuel Dreuilhe, *Mortal Embrace: Living with AIDS*, Linda Coverdale Trans., Hill and Wang, New York, (1988), p. 132.

14. 'Effects of Discrimination Outlined Before Commission', in *AIDS Policy and Law*, vol. 3, no. 5, p. 5.

15. Ibid.

16. See Gerald Dworkin, 'Autonomy and Behavior Control', *Hastings Center Report*, (1976), vol. 6, no. 1, pp. 23-8.

17. See Harry Frankfurt, 'Freedom of Will and Concept of a Person', *Journal of Philosophy*, (1971), vol. 68, pp. 5-20.

18. I wish to thank Michael Hancock for bringing this example to my attention and for extensive discussion of it.

19. Ethan A. Nadelmann, 'The Case for Legalization', *The Public Interest*, (Summer 1988), vol. 92, p. 21.

20. 'Anne Shows Ministers the Way', *Daily Express*, (January (28) 1988).

21. Consider the following example. Imagine that society decides to nurture the value of altruism. To do this it establishes policies that will give people an opportunity to act altruistically. Richard M. Titmuss, in *The Gift Relationship: From Human Blood to Social Policy*, Vintage Books, New York, (1972), has argued that exclusively voluntary blood donor systems accomplish this end.

22. For a classic discussion of this conception of the *state*, see John Stuart Mill, 'On Liberty', in *John Stuart Mill: On Liberty*, Hackett Publishing Co., Indianapolis, (1978); and R. Dworkin, 'Liberalism', in *Public and Private Morality*, Stuart Hampshire (ed), Cambridge University Press, Cambridge, (1978), pp. 113-43.

23. Nadelmann, 'The Case for Legalization', pp. 3-31.

24. Ibid, p. 17.

25. Ibid, p. 18.

26. For an excellent review article of the medical work being done on "self-esteem", see 'Self-esteem, *The Lancet*, (1988), vol. 2, pp. 943-4.

27. John Rawls, *A Theory of Justice*, Harvard University Press, Cambridge, (1971), p. 440.

28. This is not, of course, to say that it is completely within the domain of society; individual factors, including how one is raised, are also crucial. But even these are not exclusively in the domain of the individual.

29. Dreuilhe, *Mortal Embrace: Living with AIDS*, p. 34.

30. I wish to thank Morton Weinfeld (and his students) for bringing this objection to my attention.

31. Peter Finn and Taylor McNeil, 'Research Application Review: The Response of the Criminal Justice System to Bias Crime', unpublished manuscript, (October (5) 1987).

32. *Sunday Telegraph*, (June (5) 1988).

33. 'Lords Keep "Gay Clause" in Bill', *The Times*, (February (3) 1988).

34. 'Gay Sex Teaching Move is Lost', *The Times*, (December (16) 1987).

35. Digby Anderson, 'Only Discriminate', *The Times*, (February (3) 1988).

36. *Bowers* v. *Hardwick* 106 S.Ct 2841, (1986), in C. Pierce and D. VanDeVeer, *AIDS: Ethics and Public Policy*, Wadsworth Publishing Co., Belmont, Calif., (1988), p. 173.

37. Brief for Petitioner, *Bowers* v. *Hardwick* 106 S.Ct. 2841, pp. 37-8, quoted from *AIDS: Ethics and Public Policy*, p. 175.

38. It might be thought that this recent legislation is prompted strictly by AIDS and that prior to AIDS there was no discrimination against homosexuals. It is more likely that discrimination against homosexuals has been widespread and continuous. AIDS has certainly made matters worse, but more importantly it has made discrimination against homosexuals acceptable once again. It is naive to assume, that the only time discrimination exists is when it is seen by mainstream society as acceptable behavior.

39. G. B. Hastings, D. S. Leather, and A. C. Scott, 'AIDS Publicity: Some Experiences from Scotland', *British Medical Journal*, (January (3) 1987), vol. 294, no. 6563, p. 48.

40. Jeffrey A. Kelly, J. S. St. Lawrence, S. Smith, H. V. Hood and D. J. Cook, 'Medical Students' Attitudes Towards AIDS and Homosexual Patients', *Journal of Medical Education*, (July 1987), vol. 62, no. 7, pp. 549-56.

41. Ibid., p. 553.

42. Ibid.

5

The Good Society

I have argued against coercive and liberty-limiting social policy on the grounds that although the high-risk actions of gay men and IV-users are self-regarding and non-autonomous, the source of diminished autonomy has more to do with long-standing social conditions and arrangements than with particular individuals. By looking at the ways in which society may have contributed to high-risk behavior, I have moved in the direction of attributing moral responsibility for HIV/AIDS, at least for the majority of those who have the disease, to society. In the last chapter I supported a negative thesis about what social policy society ought not to develop. My position is that according to both the *strong* and *weak harm principles*, it would be wrong to impose any further harms on gay men and IV drug-users in the way of coercive social policy.

In this chapter, I consider what, if any, positive duties society has to these groups. Does society owe members of these communities anything over and above not causing them further harm? In view of the fact that the most serious harm to both gay men and IV drug-users is HIV/AIDS, a debilitating and often fatal disease, it is natural to suggest that if society does have positive duties to members of these groups, these duties should take the form of increased funding for AIDS research, education and medical and home care. Richard Mohr, in his book *Gays/Justice: A Study of Ethics, Society and Law*[1] defends this position with respect to gay men.

My strategy is as follows. To begin, I will briefly look at the argument that society owes nothing to either of these groups on the grounds that HIV/AIDS is a self-inflicted disease. If my analysis of the social forces underlying high-risk behavior is accurate, then this argument can be dismissed because it hinges on the false assumption that high-risk behavior is fully autonomous. Following this, I will look at a much more plausible and compelling argument, namely, that society owes gay men and IV-users compensation for the harm which they have inflicted on them and that it would be appropriate to compensate them in the way of increased health care. What I will not do is defend the idea that a general policy of compensation is justified when a particular group has been systematically oppressed, discriminated against and harmed by society.[2] It is an assumption of this book that compensatory policies can be morally justified and are warranted in some cases - for example, with under-represented minorities. My own position is that gay men and IV drug-users ought to be compensated financially because money is a more autonomy enhancing form of compensation.

AIDS And The Good Society

The Lifestyle Argument

In recent years, primarily because of escalating health costs, a number of people have defended the view that the costs of much health care ought to be shouldered by the unhealthy individuals who consume the care. They argue that many, if not most health problems, are the result not of factors beyond the individual's control, but of those within his control. Individuals adopt lifestyles which are hazardous to their health. That is, good health is more a function of how people live than of factors which are beyond their control. If this is a good argument, it has some interesting implications when coupled with other moral assumptions. For instance, principles of fairness are normally taken to exclude free riding. Free riding takes place when people who play fairly (follow the rules, live prudently etc.) end up shouldering the burden for those who do not. In the case of health care, in a socialist or semi-socialist system, those who live healthy and prudent lives end up carrying the health care costs of those who live unhealthy lives. Thus, the health risk takers are free riding on the more prudent low risk takers. According to this line of reasoning it is unfair that those who protect their health should have to pay for the health costs of those who throw caution to the wind with their health.

If this argument is followed through, then it may be thought to have serious implications for how people with HIV/AIDS are treated. AIDS qualifies, in the majority of cases, as a lifestyle disease. Given this and the high cost of treating persons with HIV/AIDS, many people may wish to invoke the lifestyle argument in order to undercut state-funded care of those with HIV/AIDS. In view of this, it is worthwhile to state explicitly why even if the *lifestyle argument* is a good one, it cannot be applied to persons with HIV/AIDS.

It is certainly true that individual lifestyles have a lot to do with how healthy individuals are. If someone smokes or drinks excessively, he increases his risk for a variety of serious diseases. What is less obvious, however, is that lifestyle choices are as much within the control of individuals as this argument implies. To the extent that a particular lifestyle is not chosen autonomously, the *lifestyle argument* loses any force which it might otherwise have. It would be unfair to penalize individuals for unhealthy habits, if they did not autonomously choose to have those habits or to put the matter in stronger terms, if they were manipulated into behaving in hazardous ways.

If my analysis concerning the social conditions that have fostered HIV/AIDS in the two high-risk groups is accurate, then although HIV infection may be a *lifestyle disease*, those who have it have not autonomously chosen the lifestyle which has placed them at higher risk. This point should be stressed. Given the social forces which have contributed to gay men and IV-users adopting the lifestyles which have put them at risk for HIV/AIDS it cannot be said of them that they have autonomously chosen these lifestyles. In the case of gay men there is good reason to believe that their desires for the *fast track* are socially induced, and with respect to IV-users, that were narcotics legally available, they would not be sharing injection equipment and frequenting shooting galleries. If there is reason to be sceptical about the autonomy of the lifestyle choices made by gay men and IV-users, then even if the *lifestyle argument* is plausible (which is doubtful)[3] it cannot be invoked with respect to HIV/AIDS because the crucial condition, namely, that the lifestyle be adopted autonomously, is not satisfied here. It may be that in individual instances a lifestyle is chosen autonomously, but this is not enough to justify a policy which would discriminate against persons with HIV/AIDS. Hence, if there is a positive duty to people with HIV/AIDS it is not undermined by the *lifestyle argument* even if that argument stands with respect to other health problems.

Compensatory Justice

The idea that those who have been harmed by society should be compensated for their harm is not a new one. Affirmative action and preferential hiring programs (positive discrimination) are now common. Such programs can be justified by way of two very different sorts of moral arguments. First, they can be justified on consequentialist grounds. By giving preferential treatment, for instance in hiring practices to under-represented groups, good consequences are produced. Young people need to know that members of their groups can succeed in the professions. For example, if Blacks and women hold prominent and high profile positions, they will provide others with a positive role model, and this, in turn, will encourage young Blacks and women to enter into the profession. With time, discrimination against these groups will disappear.

Second, programs of affirmative action can be justified by way of justice-based arguments. The reasoning goes as follows. Since Blacks and women have been systematically and wrongly discriminated against by society, society *owes* them compensation for the harm that they have endured. The intuition underlying this argument is that justice requires that people get what they deserve. Those who have been discriminated against deserve to be compensated and one way to compensate them is through programs of affirmative action.[4]

Much of the evidence presented in the preceding chapters suggests that compensation to gay men and IV-users is appropriate. Both groups have been wrongly discriminated against and have been harmed as a result of this discrimination. If it is conceded that those who have been harmed ought to be compensated, then it would seem to follow that gay men and IV-users ought to be compensated. The situation of members of the gay community is not dissimilar to that of individuals from groups which have benefited from anti-discriminatory policies and legislation, women and Blacks. In the US, for instance, Blacks, Hispanics and women have received preferential treatment with respect to university admissions and appointments. In these cases discrimination has been expressed in laws and social policy and has resulted in harm to members of these groups. The situation with respect to IV-users is also similar in the relevant respects. Although it is perhaps not the case that IV-users as individuals are discriminated against, it is the case that the activity in which they are engaged, narcotic use, is discriminated against. And, on at least one picture of what the *good society* is, this discrimination is wrong because it prohibits a self-regarding action. Society discriminates against IV drug-users by instituting laws which wrongfully prohibit an activity in which they wish to engage.[5] IV-users have also been harmed as a result of this discrimination. If IV drug-use were legal, the sharing of needles would not play the same role that it presently does in the IV community, and in turn, IV drug-users would not be at as high a risk as they now are.

So if we buy into the compensation argument, a case can be made on behalf of both IV-users and gay men that they are owed compensation. I propose to take as given the assumption that gay men and IV-users are deserving

candidates for compensation, and to examine the question
of what kind of compensation they are owed.[6]

A number of possibilities come to mind about what form
compensation to these two groups should take. Some
possibilities are free medical care and psychosocial
support, enhanced funding for AIDS research or financial
compensation for loss of income because of early death.
Alternatively, it may be more appropriate to abandon
altogether the idea of compensating persons in these ways
and instead to compensate them by remedying the social
forces which have put them at high risk for AIDS. A few
options will need to be considered.

What Kind of Compensation?

Before looking at what compensation would be
appropriate, it will be helpful to consider what exactly it
is for which compensation is being proposed. HIV/AIDS
is a harm which has afflicted large numbers of gay men
and IV-users; there is a correlation between it and certain
conditions within society which cannot be justified
morally. Members of both groups, then, are being
compensated for the harm which has resulted because of
unethical conditions. If the wrongful conditions existed,
(discriminatory and paternalistic laws) but did not result in
a substantial harm to either gay men or IV-users, then
there is nothing for which they need to be compensated.[7]
This point needs to be highlighted. The duty to
compensate gay men and IV drug-users who have
HIV/AIDS exists not so much because they have been
wronged, but because through these wrongs they have been
harmed. This is supported by the moral intuition that we
do not have a duty to compensate people who may have
been wronged, but who have benefited from the wrong.[8]

In addition to the harm of HIV/AIDS, gay men have been harmed in other ways. Often, because of discrimination, gay men are deterred from developing long-term intimate relationships and they may suffer from social isolation and low self-esteem. These are serious harms which should not be underestimated. But should gay men be compensated for them? The answer to this question is, I think, no and for reasons which are primarily pragmatic.

Any program of compensation is restricted by certain practical limitations.[9] The harm for which compensation is owed must be not only identifiable, but must be able to be shown to be connected to the wrongful action. Low self-esteem and social isolation are much less clearly identifiable than HIV disease and are unfortunately the products of a wide variety of conditions, some of which may and some of which may not be morally problematic. The crux of the problem is that to compensate gay men and IV drug-users for all of the harms associated with discrimination against them would be over-inclusive. That is, compensating them for loneliness, isolation and low self-esteem would involve compensating them for much which may not be a result of discrimination.

Mohr's Argument

Richard Mohr makes a compelling case for compensation to gay men in the form of government funding for patient care, especially hospice and nursing care.[10] To defend this position he argues that since society has made it impossible for gay men to form families on their own, it owes them the nurturing and protection which they would otherwise not have had. Mohr has the following to say:

> Compassion would suggest, and compensatory justice
> should require that the day-to-day care of the final-
> stage AIDS patient be provided in lieu of the care
> he would have likely had but for society's blocking
> his creation of his own family.[11]

I am sympathetic with at least the gist of Mohr's position,
that society has blocked gay men from creating their own
families. But does it follow simply from this fact that
either society owes compensation to gay men or, that if it
does owe compensation, it ought to take the form of
funding for hospice and nursing care? It will be fruitful
to look at the reasoning which leads Mohr to this
conclusion.

To begin with, according to Mohr, compensation is owed
only to gay men, since he believes that, of those who are
at greatest risk for AIDS, it is only gay men whose
opportunities to cultivate a family have been blocked.
Mohr is very specific about what kind of compensation is
appropriate and what compensation is for. Gay men are to
be compensated because they have been denied an
opportunity to cultivate a family life and they are owed
compensation which will provide them with that which
they have been denied, daily comfort and care.

This line of reasoning is fraught with problems. First of
all, it seems to entail a hidden assumption, namely, that
people have a claim on society not to put obstacles in the
way of them acquiring a family. If, however, there is such
a claim then surely it is not *only* gay men who have it.
Women who are pursuing careers are, I suppose, also
entitled to a family life. Yet society is arranged in such
a way that it is nearly impossible for them to both climb
the career ladder and participate in the pleasures of
domestic life. Should such women be compensated also?
What about the fat, the ugly and the disfigured? In a
society that prizes beauty in women those who do not

come up to par are at an extreme disadvantage in the mating market. On the reasoning to which Mohr appears to be committed, the answer to both of these questions would seem to be yes. If the main reason for compensating gay men is that they have been denied an opportunity to develop a nurturing family life, then the same reasoning should apply to anyone else who has been denied a similar opportunity.[12]

Furthermore, if the morally relevant characteristics of family life are having care, nurturing and comfort, there is no reason to think that the argument should be restricted to having an opportunity to acquire these benefits rather than to actually having them. If what people are entitled to is the benefits and not the opportunity, then it would seem to follow that all of those people who are not in possession of these benefits are entitled to them. It goes without saying that there are presently a great many old people living in dreary nursing homes who satisfy this criterion and for whom compensation ought to be forthcoming. And, of course, there are the countless number of homeless who are without care, nurturing and protection - not to mention shelter and food.

A second implicit assumption of Mohr's argument is that a) only families provide protection and care and b) all that families provide is protection and care. On the one hand, then, he overstates the case and on the other, he understates it. Consider the following.

Gay men are to be compensated because they have been denied an opportunity to develop a family to which they are entitled.[13] Mohr focuses on the protection and care with which families provide their members. Surely, though, there is neither a necessary connection between family life and care and protection nor any evidence that family life is the most efficient mechanism for providing care and protection. Mohr cites the high rate of failure among heterosexual families: 50% of non-gay marriages in the US fail. Clearly, there is something family life is not providing. There is no reason to think that care and protection are not secured in a variety of ways. Community support groups, psychotherapeutic relationships, the church and personal friendships are just a few of the venues open to people through which they can secure care and protection.

If care and protection can be secured in non-family environments, then it is by no means clear that either gay men do not already have these things or that although the state has denied gay men an opportunity to cultivate a family, it has thereby denied them comfort, nurturing and care. Empirical evidence is required to show that both of these are true in the case of gay men; that is, that gay men do not have open to them alternative sources of care and comfort and if they do not, that there is a causal connection between the absence of an opportunity to cultivate a family and having insufficient care and comfort. The problem is that there is not, on the face of it, anything about care and comfort which mark them as intimately connected with family life. Let's face it, only at the best of times and within the most ideal of families, does it make sense to ascribe to the family the kinds of benefits on which Mohr's argument would seem to hinge. And families of this calibre are very rare indeed. If, on the other hand, the issue is not so much the family, but what the family can provide, it is unclear why compensation should be restricted to hospice and nursing care. In so far as families provide care and comfort, they also provide many other things. At their best, they provide their members with self-esteem, an enriched intellectual and creative environment and emotional and financial support.

If society owes gay men compensation because it has denied them an opportunity to have a family, then there is no obvious reason why compensation should be restricted to either hospice and nursing care or gay men who have AIDS. Gay men with AIDS are only a small subset of those gay men who have been denied an opportunity to cultivate a family. If the issue is a *family life* and what it can provide, then surely everyone who has been wrongly denied these benefits ought to receive them and there is no reason to think that this class of persons consists only of gay men with AIDS. Similarly, there is no reason to think that if what gay men are to be compensated for is the loss of a family, that the form compensation takes should be restricted to hospice and nursing care.

All of this is not to say that there is not something worthwhile in Mohr's central idea, that gay men are owed compensation. Gay men are owed something from society, but not because society has denied them the opportunity to cultivate a family. They are owed something because society has pretty much restricted their sexual lifestyle options to one, the *fast track*. Because this turned out to be a hazardous way of conducting a sexual life they suffered extremely harmful consequences, the most harmful of which is AIDS. In other words, gay men are owed compensation because many of them have HIV/AIDS and they have it because of certain wrongful social conditions.

This is an important point, but one with which Mohr only flirts. When the issue is recast as one about compensation for HIV/AIDS, much of what Richard Mohr wants to claim can be claimed in a more coherent way. It makes sense to argue for compensation for gay men who have HIV/AIDS when the harm for which compensation is forthcoming is HIV/AIDS. Similarly, it is clear why hospice and nursing care are appropriate forms of compensation, when what is being compensated is HIV/AIDS.

What is less clear on this reformulation of the issue is that *only* gay men are deserving of compensation for HIV/AIDS. By looking at the social factors which have fostered HIV/AIDS in the two highest risk groups, it can be seen that just as gay men have been afflicted with the disease because of certain wrongful social conditions, so have IV drug-users. In both instances social conditions which cannot be justified morally have fostered the disease. In view of this, IV drug-users would seem to be just as entitled to compensation as are gay men.

Compensation in the Form of Health Care

Knowing that gay men and IV drug-users who have HIV/AIDS are owed compensation does not get us any further ahead in answering the following question: What form should compensation take? In my analysis of Mohr's position, I showed that it does not make sense for compensation to gay men to take the form of increased funding for hospice and nursing care if what you are compensating them for is a denied opportunity to have a family. It does, however, make sense to provide them with these benefits if they are being compensated for HIV/AIDS.

But after careful consideration of the social conditions which have fostered the disease, funding for hospice and nursing care is much less appealing as a form of compensation. At least in part, what I have shown is that gay men and IV-users have had their autonomy severely diminished by society. Because the set of options from which they could choose was reduced and by means which could not be justified morally, they had certain desires induced and were manipulated into making choices which may well not reflect their autonomous wishes. In view of this, it would seem only right that any compensation which is owed to them reflect a concern with autonomy. That is, compensation ought to be autonomy enhancing rather than autonomy diminishing.

Is funding for hospice and nursing care autonomy enhancing? This question can be answered only relatively. Mohr vividly describes the following unfortunate scenario.

> One of the sadder moral side effects of the AIDS crisis is the number of men, stricken in their prime and deprived of medical insurance by forced unemployment, who have had to return to their frequently bewildered mothers and alien environments to be nursed through the final months of their suffering. Effectively denied the possibility of creating his own nurturing family, the son experiences the final humiliation of being treated again as a child, accepted, if at all, not for himself, but in spite of himself.[14]

Although Mohr is not explicit about what exactly it is about this scenario that is morally offensive, certainly one of his concerns is with the autonomy of the person with AIDS. This is clear from his description of the final humiliation of the person with AIDS, namely, being treated again as a child. There is no doubt that this scenario is both humiliating and autonomy diminishing for gay men. And this final insult to autonomy is certainly inexcusable in view of the long-term offence to autonomy which gay men have endured. Why suppose, though, that government-funded hospice and nursing care will change this?

Autonomy and Government-Funded Hospice and Nursing Care

Some reduction in autonomy is inevitable with the final stage AIDS patient because he is very ill. This is not, however, to say that their autonomy status cannot be improved. Even though government-funded hospice and nursing care will give gay men an alternative to returning to their parents, it does not increase their sense of control over their lives. Society continues to dictate the terms under which they will die. Medical care is distributed either on a nationalized state-funded system or through an individual consumer pays system. It will be worthwhile to consider the proposal that gay men and IV-users be compensated for HIV/AIDS in view of these two mechanisms for distributing health care.[15]

Need-Based Health Care
Ideally in a nationalized system, full health care benefits would be provided to people with HIV/AIDS. Were such a system to exist the question of compensating gay men and IV-users with health care would not arise. Since gay men and IV drug-users would already receive state-funded health care, they could not be compensated with it. In such a system, compensation would have to take another form. But, in these times of scarce medical resources few health care systems can afford to cover the costs of *all* health care needs.[16] Most of the major collectivist systems are plagued with serious economic problems and have been forced to cut back.

Consider the following report about the presently troubled British health care system. In the late eighties, Birmingham hospitals were ordered by regional health authorities to stop taking on new dialysis patients because of financial problems. According to the British Kidney

Patients Association 37,000 people have died in the last thirteen years because they could not get dialysis. It is not only the elderly who are being denied access to dialysis. Elizabeth Ward, president of the Association, claims that doctors make life and death decisions on the "basis of a patient's social status, denying treatment to people who are jobless, alcoholic or who cannot speak English".[17] Nor is dialysis the only treatment to which people do not have access or for which they must wait long periods of time. According to this report, approximately 700,000 people are waiting for elective surgery such as hip replacements and cataract surgery. Some have waited for as long as five years.[18]

The British National Health Service was until recently one of the best health care systems available. Now plagued with financial problems it has difficulty meeting the health care needs of those who depend on it. The situation is not much better in Canada where health care is also distributed according to collectivist principles. Canadian hospitals regularly experience bed shortages and there are long waiting lists for medical tests and surgery.

In view of the financial problems that can plague nationalized health care systems, there is no reason to think that persons with HIV/AIDS will be immune to experiencing the effects of cutbacks. This is an especially threatening possibility because the costs of AIDS are high and those who have the disease stigmatized. Even within a nationalized system there is reason to believe that the medical costs for persons with HIV/AIDS will not be covered completely and hence that there may still be room for *preferential health care*. Would compensation in the form of health care be desirable in these circumstances?

The moral intuition underlying collectivized medicine is that medical care ought to be distributed on the basis of need. To compensate gay men and IV drug-users with *preferential health care* would entail introducing a new criterion for the distribution of health care. Namely, health care on the basis of desert.[19] It is not at all clear, though, that 1) health care according to need and 2) health care according to desert are compatible within one and the same system. What are the implications of introducing 2) into a system in which 1) prevails?

This scenario is fraught with problems. The main problem is one that has to do with the demands of consistency. If both 1) and 2) are at work within any given system, and if there is a greater demand for health care than the system can provide, there will be people, other than gay men and IV-users with HIV/AIDS, who will wish to make a claim to health care by invoking the criterion of desert; and their claim may be well founded. Once a move is made in the direction of the criterion of desert, there is no morally relevant reason to restrict desert with the caveat that only those with HIV/AIDS deserve enriched health care.

It may be that people who have been victimized by other sorts of social arrangements ought also to qualify for health care under the desert criterion. On the face of the matter, it would seem to be morally arbitrary to exclude them. Why should gay men and IV drug-users receive health care on the desert criterion, but, for example, not the homeless and the abused? A strong argument could be marshalled for both the homeless and the abused by showing that they have been harmed by social arrangements and hence deserve enhanced health care. Once a new criterion, affording new benefits, is introduced into an impoverished system there are going to be others vying for the rewards of that criterion and there is no obvious way of excluding them.

Health care distributors would be saddled with the insurmountable task of having to decide among different deserving factions. Do persons with HIV/AIDS have a stronger claim to health care than the homeless or women who have also experienced discrimination? But this would not exhaust the challenge to health care distributors. Sometimes those who have the strongest desert-based claim to health care would not have the strongest need-based claim to it. Put differently, those who deserve health care according to the desert criterion may not be among the neediest of the sick. The crux of the problem is that these two criteria represent two distinct and incommensurable moral paradigms for distributing health care resources.

The consequences of providing desert-based health benefits to *only* gay men and IV-users who have HIV/AIDS would be disastrous. Although they may die in more pleasant surroundings, the stigma and resentment which they already experience may well increase. Not only would they be held responsible for spreading AIDS, but under the proposed revised system, they would probably also be held responsible for robbing others of scarce medical resources.[20]

Ability-Based Health Care

In a system such as the one in place in the US, where the primary criterion for distribution of health care resources is *each according to his ability* a different set of problems emerge. This is not to say that the same problems associated with introducing a new and divergent criterion into a system would not also exist, because they would. But there are others. For one thing, although need-based distribution is not entirely foreign to the US, it is rare and remains controversial. The indigent and the old receive health benefits from both state and federal governments. Thus, the neediest members of society are provided with state-funded health care.

Because the guiding principle for distribution of health care in the US is ability to pay, those who receive health care on the basis of need do not receive it because they have a moral claim on society to provide them with it.[21] They receive it because society is good enough to give it to them; society acts altruistically in this case. This may have the consequence of marking the recipient of state-funded health care as to some extent a less than full member of society, someone who is unable to take care of himself and who because of this must be taken care of by the state. Though the indigent and old are perhaps better off with respect to health care than they would be without this provision, they pay a high price for it. They are by no means better off with respect to personal autonomy; they are told what services they can receive and where they can receive them. But even worse, they pay a high price in personal self-esteem. It would be difficult to have self-esteem in a society that values emotional and financial independence, when one is ill and can neither take care of oneself practically nor financially. In the US, those who receive state-funded health care, the indigent and the old, are not much better off than children who must depend upon their parents. With respect to how they are viewed in society, they may well be worse off. Children, after all, are not expected to be emotionally and financially independent.

Mohr thinks that gay men ought to receive state-funded hospice and nursing care so that they may die as dignified adults, free from the humiliating experience of having to return to their parents. Mohr's position, though well intended, is naive. Even though the justification for funding their health care expenses is different from the justification for funding the expenses of the old and the indigent, gay men and IV drug-users would inevitably be viewed and treated in much the same way as the old and indigent. Given the loss to self-esteem and autonomy already endured by gay men, this proposal would do little more than saddle them with more of the same kind of harm which they have already had to endure.[22] Still, a criterion for choosing among different forms of compensation can be rescued from this analysis. Namely, that whatever form of compensation is chosen, it should enhance the autonomy of gay men and IV-users.

There is more to dying with dignity and self-esteem than simply being provided with certain medical amenities. Looking at how health care is delivered in the US and keeping in mind the extent to which gay men have been discriminated against there, it is not difficult to see that there is not much difference, from the point of view of gay men, between having to return to one's parents for nurturing and care or receiving it from the state. In both cases one may be, given the particular people involved, dependent upon one's oppressors.[23]

Compensation and Individual Autonomy

There is one overriding reason why providing medical care as a form of compensation is not a particularly autonomy enhancing way of compensating gay men and IV drug-users, or anyone else for that matter. One very sure way of enhancing someone's autonomy is to open the field of significant options from which they can choose.[24] To enhance autonomy give individuals more *real* choices. In this way, the likelihood that an option will be available to them which is consistent with what they want for themselves is increased. By increasing the number of options available to persons, they are provided with the opportunity to be self-determining.

Compensating people with enriched health care does not enhance autonomy because it does not enlarge the sphere of options available to them. At most, it gives them one option which may not have been available to them before compensation was proffered. The problem is that compensating people in this way dictates the content of the compensation. It goes without saying that not all gay men and IV-users are going to want the same thing. Some may decide that they want to be cared for by their lovers or families; others may wish to forego altogether the final stage of AIDS and instead opt for suicide and still others may have a strong desire to donate money to the Gay Men's Christian League or to the Cancer Research Foundation. Those who do want health care may want something other than what traditional medicine has to offer; they may be interested in acupuncture or homeopathic medicine.[25]

It might be argued that at least some of my reservations about health care as a form of compensation can be accommodated by a voucher system.[26] Gay men and IV drug-users who have HIV/AIDS could be given health care vouchers which they could use at the health care institution of their choice. There is no doubt that such a system would be more autonomy enhancing than a system which dictates exactly who is to deliver health care and when. But there is also no doubt that this system would not provide much redress for those people who are not seeking health care at all or who would rather receive alternative therapies through non-conventional sources. More importantly, though, compensation in the form of health care conveys an extremely paternalistic message. It implies that people are not able to make responsible choices, that they would not act in their own best interest. By dictating the terms of compensation, namely health care, the voucher system fails to maximize options.

These examples provide just a few reasons why compensation in the form of health care may not be the best idea. The crux of the matter is that there are enough people who would choose to be compensated in a different way to justify finding an alternative mode of compensation. If all gay men and IV drug-users could be counted on to have uniform desires with respect to the issue of health care and compensation, there would not be a problem in compensating them in this way. But gay men and IV-users are no different from the rest of the population in this respect; they are not uniform in what they desire.

It is important to compensate gay men and IV-users in a way that will enhance their autonomy because they have already endured a decrease in autonomy. The best way to do this is to give them compensation in the form of money. Money will give them the wherewithal to do what they want. It will allow them to purchase the kind of health care they want, to support famine relief or cancer research or to leave money to a poor relative. As a means of compensation it respects them as autonomous agents because it respects their human capacity to make choices.

Some Practical Considerations

There are a number of practical considerations that would need to be addressed before such a program of compensation could be instituted. For example, who exactly should be compensated? Everyone with HIV/AIDS? If so, then some people would be compensated even though they do not deserve it.[27] Not everyone who has HIV/AIDS is either gay or an IV drug-user. Still, it might be that for administrative reasons HIV antibody status is the most efficient criterion of eligibility for compensation.[28] Although identifying IV drug-users would be a simple matter, the same is not true for gay men. There is no clear-cut characteristic by which the latter could be identified. And the kind of process that would allow administrators to discern whether or not someone is gay would be far too invasive to privacy to invoke.

A criterion that would result in compensating more people than those who actually deserve it (over-inclusive) is preferable to one that compensates fewer people than those who deserve it (under-inclusive). If the duty to compensate gay men and IV drug-users is taken seriously, then it is more important that all of those who are thought to be deserving of compensation receive it, than that some who do not deserve it, receive it. The problem of over-inclusiveness is not unique to this proposal for compensation. Affirmative action programs in the US face the same difficulty. For example, a program that targets Blacks wants to confer benefits on underprivileged Blacks who have suffered from discrimination; it is not aimed at middle-class Blacks who may have benefited from all the best schools. But there is just no effective way to exclude them. To try to do so might entail excluding those who are deserving.[29]

Another practical point that needs to be considered is who should receive how much money. Should those with full-blown AIDS receive more than those with HIV infection? AIDS is a worse harm than HIV infection. It is more debilitating and people die from it. The issue is a bit more complicated than this since although not everyone with HIV infection may end up with full-blown cases of AIDS a good portion of them do. Thus, HIV infection is viewed by many as a death sentence.

One way to approach this question is to look at the potential earnings someone with HIV/AIDS would have were he to live a full and productive life. This could be calculated on the basis of the average earnings of members of that society. At the time that HIV infection is diagnosed individuals could begin to collect compensation. They might receive an annual fixed amount which would continue until they die. Those who live longest would, on this model, receive more compensation than those who die early.

This differentiation in amount of money persons with HIV/AIDS would receive may seem to be unfair. Given the grounds for compensation, namely, the correlation between wrongful social conditions and HIV/AIDS, a fair distribution would give to each recipient an amount which corresponds to the degree to which his encounter with HIV/AIDS can be accounted for by these conditions. Although there is a correlation between certain social conditions and developing HIV/AIDS, there is not a specific correlation between the severity of one's illness and the relevant social conditions. Because of this, there is no way to assess, on the basis of illness alone, the extent to which the severity of any particular person's encounter with the disease is due to the oppressive social context. Obtaining the information needed to answer this question would require extensive and highly intrusive interviews with potential recipients. The costs to individual self-esteem, personal integrity and autonomy entailed by such interviews may be viewed by many as too high a price to pay for compensation.

A distribution of compensation benefits which would give to each exactly what he deserves, according to the grounds for compensation, cannot be had. The advantage of compensating people annually is that it would offset some of the problems inherent to compensating people with money. For instance, one objection to compensating people with money, especially IV drug-users, is that they are not autonomous enough to make good use of it.[30] If a *junkie* is simply handed $30,000, he will spend it satisfying his non-autonomous thirst for narcotics. Earlier I argued against the position that *only* autonomous desires ought to be respected mainly on the grounds that if this avenue were taken it would undermine the capacity to be autonomous.[31] Some of the considerations raised in that discussion apply as well to the present one. Respecting persons as autonomous agents often requires that they be allowed to do not only what they autonomously wish to do, but also what, in more reflective moments, they would not endorse doing. It is only through coming to be autonomous that people develop essential autonomy skills.

IV drug-users are often from poverty-stricken backgrounds, from which they have little hope of escape. In many cases narcotic use is inspired by the hopelessness of these very circumstances. It may be that the prospect of a less impoverished future, which would accompany annual compensation benefits, would make many IV drug-users reconsider their drug habit. They might, knowing that the next year promises future benefits, seek treatment or at least be more prudent in how they take drugs (for instance, they might be more cautious with respect to needle-sharing). These options would be more feasible for them, if treatment programs were readily available and narcotics legally accessible. The prospect of a decent future, which most people take for granted, is a powerful incentive for prudent living.

Although distributing compensation in the way that I recommend may decrease narcotic use, this should not be viewed as the goal of my proposal. It is important to bear in mind that narcotic use is a self-regarding action and the harm involved a self-inflicted one. The bottom line is that in the *good society* people must be permitted such liberties.

Other Obligations

Duties to gay men and IV drug-users who have HIV/AIDS do not rest with compensation. In addition to direct compensation to those with HIV/AIDS there are obligations to both gay men and IV drug-users to right the wrongs which have conspired to put them at risk for HIV/AIDS. For gay men this would require immediate removal of all discriminatory laws and policies as well as a campaign designed to promote homosexuality as a legitimate lifestyle option. For IV drug-users paternalistic policies and laws which prohibit narcotic use must be dismantled and in their place legal access to narcotics instituted. Also because of the severe curtailment of autonomy experienced by both gay men and IV-users some further consideration of how society might enhance their autonomy is needed.[32]

Education

Education programs are one of the more autonomy enhancing avenues available to society designed to slow the spread of the virus. But not all education programs fare equally well with respect to individual autonomy. Many sacrifice respect for the person in the name of effectiveness. Particular caution needs to be exercised when adopting education policies that are effective because they pressure people or frighten them into changing their behavior. It needs to be borne in mind that behavior can be changed in a variety of ways, some of which will promote autonomy and some of which won't.[33] On the definition of *autonomy* which I gave in Chapter 3[34] an autonomous person has to identify with his desires, endorse them as his own. For a person to be autonomous in this sense he has to have not only a first-order desire for x, but also a second-order desire about his desire for x. So, for example, if a desire for safer sex is to qualify as an autonomous one, then the person who desires safer sex must have, in addition to this desire, a second-order desire to desire the desire for safer sex. When both first and second-order desires are present, it is much more likely that the person concerned actually endorses being the kind of person who has that particular desire. In other words, it is more likely that the desire is an autonomous one.

In the *good society*, there is a presumption in favor of the autonomous person and hence autonomous decision-making and autonomous desire formation. Respect for persons requires that they be provided with the opportunities they need to exercise their capacity to be autonomous and to formulate autonomous desires. This does not mean that society is obliged to refrain altogether from trying to influence what desires individuals come to have. But it does mean that only some forms of influence will be morally justifiable.

Consider an example taken from outside of AIDS issues. Suppose that a man who is a chronic cigarette smoker and who values his autonomy wants to quit smoking. To this end, he can avail himself of a number of different therapies, all of which promise relief from the desire for nicotine. He can take pills, subject himself to shock therapy or aversion therapy, or he can contract for ten weeks of psychotherapy. Our addict is interested not only in quitting his habit, but doing so in a way that is respectful of his autonomy. He opts for psychotherapy. The *talking cure*, unlike the others, will allow him to come to identify with the desire to not smoke.[35]

Just as different forms of therapy are more or less autonomy enhancing, so are different methods of educating people about HIV/AIDS and effecting behavior change in those who persist in high-risk behavior. To fully recognize this point, it is important that we be weaned from the idea that behavior must be changed no matter what the cost and put in its place the idea that behavior should be changed in a way that respects and promotes individual autonomy.[36] It is not the case that education of any kind is autonomy enhancing.

Harvey Fineberg in an article entitled "Education to Prevent HIV/AIDS: Prospects and Obstacles"[37] discusses the various problems that different education measures face as well as what educational formats are most promising. He speaks highly of the *educational interventions* adopted by the gay community in San Francisco and New York. Among those he mentions are community outreach programs, distribution of educational literature, media campaigns, telephone hotlines and peer discussion and support groups that reinforce changes in behavior.[38] Although Fineberg praises these endeavors, he cautions that they may not be effective enough and may need to be supplemented.

> If there is to be a widespread and persistent shift in behavior related to sex and drugs, it must be grounded in a shift in social norms.[39]

The idea, as I understand it, is that the way to complement, perhaps reinforce individual efforts to change behavior, is to make some behavior socially acceptable and others unacceptable. Social norms can be used to encourage safer behavior. This theme is echoed and developed by Norbert Gilmore in a paper entitled "Sex, AIDS and Cultural Change."[40] The measures which Fineberg seems to flirt with are strongly defended by Gilmore.

> Education at a population level and counselling at an individual level are essential. When successful,

safe behavior must be reinforced so that it will be sustained. There are three approaches to change this behavior: fear; health promotion models to change individual attitudes, knowledge and behavior; and peer pressure. Each of these approaches appear to be operative now, and each will be essential if the spread of HIV is to be stopped.[41]

Gilmore suggests not only that social norms be modified in order to sustain behavior change, but also that fear and peer pressure be put to work on this task. There are a couple of objections to this tack.

A wide range of different and significant opportunities is important for individual autonomy. Programs which aim to reduce options are, of course, problematic for autonomy. This is so even when the options which are being taken away by revising social norms are ones which are harmful to individuals. If smoking becomes socially unacceptable, as many would have it, such that it is no longer a real option, then the smoker's liberty is diminished even though his health may be much improved. He has fewer real options from which to choose; hence less autonomy. But even more problematic is the lack of respect for individual autonomy that these tactics betray.

Promoting behavior change and inducing desires conducive to good health through fear and social pressure do not allow people to come to identify with the new desires and behavior. These methods do little more than manipulate people into adopting behavior which is either thought by others to be in their best interest or might be agreed by all to be in their best interest. In either case, the methods used are repugnant from the point of view of autonomy.

Take the case of social pressure. Suppose that anonymous sex becomes a thing of the past. No longer can a gay man (or for that matter a heterosexual man or woman) even express a desire for anonymous sex, let alone secure it. Social pressure has made this impossible. There are two reasons why this is problematic. First, a person with an anonymous sex desire is no longer at liberty to do something which he may want to do. Because of this, his liberty is interfered with. He has fewer real options than he might otherwise have. In so far as his desire for anonymous sex is an autonomous one, his autonomy may also be hampered. In Chapter 3, I argued that there is convincing evidence that, in general, the desire for anonymous sex is not autonomous. This is not to say that it could not be autonomous. In a world where gay men had a wide variety of sexual lifestyle options from which to choose, they might well come to formulate an autonomous desire for anonymous sex. For example, this might be so if they had open to them the same panoply of options open to heterosexual men: long-term monogamy, sequential monogamy, long-term sexual intimacies combined with short-term affairs, or long-term sexual intimacy combined with anonymous sexual encounters, or just anonymous sex or, some combination of these over a life-time. Heterosexual men, though perhaps under some social pressure to marry, nonetheless have a variety of sexual lifestyle options from which to choose. This places them in the ideal situation of being able to choose one which is concert with their self-conception. They can experiment with any number of options until they find one which is well suited to them. And they might well opt for anonymous sex or some combination of it with long-term intimacy. In other words, the panoply of sexual lifestyle options open to heterosexual men provides them with a better chance of formulating an autonomous desire for one or more of them.

The same has not been true for gay men. Discrimination and fear of social rejection and aggression have conspired to reduce their options to one, impersonal sex with fleeting and often unsuccessful attempts at long-term intimacy. When there is only one real option available, it is difficult to desire anything other than it and the context is ripe for adaptive preference formation. For gay men the choice may be more or less impersonal sex or no sex and this can scarcely be said to qualify as a choice. Were the situation different, were there a variety of sexual lifestyle options available to gay men, they would no doubt display as much variation in sexual lifestyle preferences as do heterosexual men. Some would come to identify with monogamy, some with sequential monogamy and some with impersonal sex. Because the number and variety of options available to people is important for autonomy, programs which seek to change behavior by reducing options threaten autonomy.

I am not advocating that gay men choose high-risk impersonal sex. However, I do think that autonomy considerations demand that it remain an option. It may be that most gay men would find it an unattractive option precisely because of the risks associated with it and that few would come to identify with it because of this. This scenario is all the more likely if other substantive sexual lifestyle options are made available to them. If one of the main reasons why gay men choose frequent impersonal sex is because their options are limited to *this* or *no* sex, then it makes sense that by increasing the significant options they have in this arena, they would also be provided with the opportunity to choose autonomously in favor of other low-risk sexual lifestyles.

Gay men may change their behavior as a result of fear and peer pressure, but this change would not be an autonomous one. Paradoxically, these methods simply mimic those which have led to high-risk behavior in the first place. With respect to high-risk behavior, options were reduced until there was no option but impersonal sex. Now with respect to safer sex practices, the suggestion is that gay men be coerced into safe sex by reducing their options. They will again be left with a *this* or *nothing* option. There is little evidence that in addition to eliminating unsafe sex as a real option, new options will be introduced.

Education programs that aim at changing behavior through fear and social pressure are morally problematic because they deny individuals a crucial opportunity to change their behavior and desires in ways which respect their uniquely human capacity to be autonomous. Forcing people to modify their behavior by leaving them no real options fails to respect them because it denies them an opportunity to make a choice about a significant matter, namely, how they conduct their sexual lives.

Concluding Remarks

Society has both positive and negative duties to gay men and IV drug-users with HIV/AIDS. These include the negative duty to not establish laws and policies which will further interfere with the liberty and autonomy of gay men and IV drug-users and, of course, to remove those which presently do infringe on their liberty. But society's duties to gay men and IV drug-users are not restricted to negative duties. If my analysis is accurate many of the gay men and IV drug-users who have HIV/AIDS have it because of certain social conditions which do not have to exist and which do not befit the *good society*. Poverty, racism, discrimination against homosexuals and intolerance of different life-plans are social conditions which cannot do anything but harm people. AIDS is perhaps a greater harm than anyone anticipated. But this fact does not diminish social responsibility for it. Social conditions which are recognizably harmful were allowed to persist with little concern for those who suffered because of them. AIDS makes it impossible to continue to ignore these problems and our responsibility for them. But AIDS also gives us an opportunity to amend some of this harm. Our positive duties go beyond pecuniary compensation, which is in a sense only a token gesture. Society must begin to take seriously the claim of *all* individuals to formulate and act on their conceptions of the *good life*. This requires more than just removing obstacles; it also requires that people be given real options.

NOTES

1. Richard D. Mohr, *Gays/Justice: A Study of Ethics, Society and Law*, Columbia University Press, New York, (forthcoming).

2. See Richard Wasserstrom, 'A Defense of Programs of Preferential Treatment', *National Forum*, vol. 58, no. 1, (1978), pp. 15-18.

3. See for example, Daniel I. Wikler, 'Persuasion and Coercion for Health: Ethical Issues in Government Efforts to Change Lifestyles', *Milbank Memorial Fund Quarterly/Health and Society*, (1978), vol. 56, no. 3, p. 303.

4. As Mill tried to show in Chapter 5 of *Utilitarianism*, although perhaps not as perspicuously as one would like, the concept of *desert* is not without utility and can be incorporated into the consequentialist scheme of things. John Stuart Mill, *Utilitarianism*, Oskar Piest (ed.), Bobbs-Merrill, Indianapolis, (1957).

5. Such a prohibition can be viewed as discriminatory because other equally harmful self-regarding actions are not prohibited: smoking, excessive alcohol consumption and sky diving.

6. It has been suggested to me that because society did not *intend* that gay men and IV drug-users develop HIV/AIDS and could not have foreseen this as a consequence of what it did, it ought not to be taken to have duties of compensation. It is important to note that although society did not intend that gay men and IV drug-users develop HIV/AIDS, nor could they have foreseen this, it did perform actions (discriminatory and paternalistic legislation, intolerance, racism) which it would be naive to think would not result in harm to members of these two groups. At the very least, it has failed to take into account the effect of its actions on people in these two communities. In some cases the harms caused by certain policies are quite obvious. Laws which prohibit narcotics make quality control impossible and IV drug-users are, in turn, harmed by bad drugs. A variety of harms were foreseeable and possibly intended, but they were dismissed as either unimportant or necessary consequences of justified policies. If we grant that some harms were foreseen and possibly intended, and that the actions from which these harms came about were morally wrong, then it is neither morally, nor legally counter-intuitive, to hold society responsible for the harms which it did not intend, but which were consequences of the wrongful

action. The legal maxim take your victim as you find him applies here. If we admit that gay men and IV drug-users have been harmed and then ask who should pay for that harm, surely the answer is not gay men and IV drug-users, but rather those who have performed the wrongful actions that resulted in the harm. I wish to thank Margaret Somerville, Harold Bursztajn and Andy Orkin for discussion on this point.

7. This is not to say that we do not have a duty to remove the wrongful conditions.

8. It is worth noting that this notion of *compensation* is not reflected in the law where compensation may be awarded for a wrong from which no harm is forthcoming or even a wrong which produces a benefit. For example, a Jehovah's witness whose life is saved by a blood transfusion which she declines, has been wronged - but has benefitted from the wrong (she lives) and may legally be entitled to compensation. In part, the issue here turns on how we understand what constitutes *harm* and *benefit*. The cases I am concerned with are more in line with compensation to a group such as Blacks, where it is the conjunction of a *wrong* plus a *harm* which warrants compensation. I am grateful to Margaret Somerville for discussion of this point.

9. See James W. Nickel, 'Classification by Race in Compensatory Programs' *Philosophical Issues in Law: Cases and Materials*, Kenneth Kipnis (ed.), Prentice-Hall, New Jersey, (1977), pp. 235-40.

10. Mohr, *Gays/Justice: A Study of Ethics, Society and Law*, p. 238.

11. Ibid.

12. Although women who fall into the categories I describe are not legally prevented from forming families in the way that gay men are, there are obstacles of a more practical kind which stand in the way of them cultivating a family life. From a moral point of view there is no reason to restrict the discussion of this issue to legal obstacles.

13. Mohr may be adopting a legal conception of compensation, but if so he needs to make this explicit and to explain it.

14. Mohr, *Gays/Justice: A Study of Ethics, Society and Law*, p. 238.

15. I should note that these considerations are not relevant to Mohr's position. His main focus is AIDS in America.

16. High-technology medicine and an expanding elderly population have made medical costs rise in recent years. For a discussion of the moral and policy implications of these changes see Daniel Callahan, *Setting Limits*, Simon and Schuster, New York, 1987.

17. Nicholas Regush, 'The Kidney Patients Britain Allows to Die', *Montreal Gazette*, (May (22) 1988).

18. Ibid.

19. To say that gay men and IV-users are owed health care as compensation is tantamount to saying that we ought to fund their health care because they have been harmed and hence *deserve* compensation.

20. This raises a problem which I do not address here, but which ought to be addressed. How much of society's resources ought to go to AIDS? Correspondingly, what criterion should be used to decide this? It is important to bear in mind that funds directed to AIDS research may be funds which other worthy causes, such as cancer research, do not receive.

21. In a collectivized system, such as Britain's and Canada's, health care is thought to be a *right* and it is experienced by people as such.

22. There are other problems with using health care as a form of compensation which I do not go into here, but which would be interesting to look at. One question that needs to be addressed is whether or not health care is the kind of good which ought to be immune from being used as a form of compensation. This would be so, for instance, if one believes that health care ought to be distributed *only* on the basis of need. Also, if one believes this then there might be practical reasons for not using it to compensate those who are owed compensation. Doing so may just prolong the time during which the ability-based criterion is in place.

23. See for example, Emmanuel Dreuilhe, *Mortal Embrace: Living with AIDS*, Linda Coverdale Trans. Hill and Wang, New York, (1988).

24. See Joseph Raz, *The Morality of Freedom*, Clarendon Press, Oxford, (1986), Chapter 14, pp. 369-95.

25. I am grateful to Margaret Duckett for this point.

26. I wish to thank Harold Bursztajn for discussion of this point.

27. It may turn out after analysis that other people with AIDS are also deserving of compensation - hemophiliacs and children for example.

28. See James W. Nickel, 'Classification by Race in Compensatory Programs', pp. 235-40.

29. Of course, this would have to be reconsidered if the make-up of the disease changes dramatically.

30. I wish to thank Harold Bursztajn for bringing this objection to my attention.

31. See Chapter 4, p. 114-16.

32. Stated-funded access to psychoanalysis might be warranted for this purpose.

33. See Gerald Dworkin, 'Autonomy and Behavior Control', *Hastings Center Report*, (1976), vol. 6, no. 1, pp. 23-8.

34. See Chapter 3.

35. It does this by increasing self-knowledge and self-awareness.

36. It may be that autonomous behavior change is more long-lasting than non-autonomous behavior change. This would be a valuable area for research.

37. Harvey V. Fineberg 'Education to Prevent AIDS: Prospects and Obstacles', *Science*, (February 1988), vol. 239, no. 5, pp. 592-6.

38. Ibid., p. 594.

39. Ibid.

40. Norbert Gilmore, 'Sex, AIDS and Cultural Change', *The Sex Information and Education Council of Canada Journal*, (1988), vol. 3, no. 4, pp. 3-13.

41. Ibid., p. 9.

Works Cited

(August 9 1987) 'AIDS: A Global Assessment', *Los Angeles Times*, supplement, 16 pgs

Altman, Dennis (1986) *AIDS in the Mind of America*, New York, Anchor Press/Doubleday

Altman, Lawrence (February 5 1989) 'Who's Stricken and How: AIDS Pattern is Shifting', *New York Times*

Anderson, Digby (February 3 1988) 'Only Discriminate', *The Times*

(January 28 1988) 'Anne Shows Ministers the Way', *Daily Express*

Anonymous (December 7 1987) 'A Painful Struggle to Beat The Odds', *Globe and Mail*, Toronto

Bartky, Sandra (1979) 'On Psychological Oppression', in *Philosophy and Women*, S. Bishop and M. Weinzweig, Belmont, Calif., Wadsworth Publishing Co., pp. 33-41

Bayer, Ronald (1986) 'AIDS, Power and Reason', *The Milbank Quarterly*, vol. 64, Suppl. 1, pp. 168-82

Beauchamp, Dan E. (1986) 'Morality and the Health of the Body Politic', *Hastings Center Report*, vol. 16, no. 6, pp. 30-6

_____ (1983) 'Public Health as Social Justice', in *Moral Problems in Medicine*, R. Macklin and S. Gorovitz, eds, New Jersey, Prentice-Hall

Bell, Alan P. and Martin S. Weinberg (1978) *Homosexualities: A Study of Diversity Among Men and Women*, New York, Simon and Schuster

Black, David (1985) *The Plague Years: A Chronicle of AIDS, the Epidemic of our Times*, New York, Simon and Schuster

Blendon, Robert J. and Karen Donelan (1988) 'Discrimination Against People with AIDS', *The New England Journal of Medicine*, vol. 319, no. 15, pp. 1022-6

Bursztajn, Harold, R. T. Feinbloom, R. M. Hamm and A. Bradsky (1983) *Medical Choices, Medical Chances: How Patients, Families and Physicians can Cope With Uncertainty*, New York, Delta/Seymour Lawrence

Callahan, Daniel (1987) *Setting Limits*, New York, Simon and Schuster

Centers for Disease Control (1981) 'Pneumocystis Pneumonia - Los Angeles', *Morbidity, Mortality Weekly Report*, vol. 30, pp. 250-2

_____ (March 10 1985) *AIDS Weekly Surveillance Report*

Des Jarlais, Don C., Samuel R. Friedman and David Strug (1986) 'AIDS and Needle Sharing Within the IV-Drug Use Subculture', in *The Social Dimensions of AIDS: Method and Theory*, D. A. Feldman and T. M. Johnson, eds, New York, Praeger, pp. 111-25

Dreuilhe, Emmanuel (1988) *Mortal Embrace: Living With AIDS*, Linda Coverdale Trans., New York, Hill and Wang

Dworkin, Gerald (1976) 'Autonomy and Behavior Control', *Hastings Center Report*, vol. 6, no. 1, pp. 23-8

Dworkin, Ronald (1978) 'Liberalism', in *Public and Private Morality*, Stuart Hampshire, ed., Cambridge, Cambridge University Press, pp. 113-43

(March 23 1988) 'Effects of Discrimination Outlined Before Commission', *AIDS Policy and Law*, vol. 3, no. 5, pp. 5-6

Elster, Jon (1983) *Sour Grapes: Studies in the Subversion of Rationality*, Cambridge, Cambridge University Press

Feinberg, Joel (1986) *Harm to Self*, New York, Oxford University Press

Fineberg, Harvey V. (1988) 'Education to Prevent AIDS: Prospects and Obstacles', *Science*, vol. 239, no. 5, pp. 592-6

_____ (1988) 'The Social Dimensions of AIDS', *Scientific American*, vol. 259, no. 4. pp. 128-34

Finn, Peter and Taylor McNeil (1987) 'Research Application Review: The Response of the Criminal Justice System to Bias Crime', unpublished manuscript

Fitzgerald, Frances (July 28 1986) 'A Reporter at Large - The Castro-II', *New Yorker*, pp. 45-63

Frankfurt, Harry (1971) 'Freedom of Will and Concept of a Person', *Journal of Philosophy*, vol. 68, pp. 5-20

Freedman, Benjamin (1981) 'Competence, Marginal and Otherwise: Concepts and Ethics', *International Journal of Law and Psychiatry*, vol. 4, pp. 53-72

Friedland, Gerald H. and Robert S. Klein (1987) 'Transmission of the Human Immunodeficiency Virus', *New England Journal of Medicine*, vol. 317, no. 18, pp. 1125-35

Friedman, S. R., D. C. Des Jarlais and J. L. Sotheran (1986) 'AIDS Health Education for Intravenous Drug Users', *Health Education Quarterly*, vol. 13, no. 4, pp. 383-93

Bibliographical References

Friedman, S. R., D. C. Des Jarlais, J. L. Sotheran, J. Garber, H. Cohen and D. Smits (1987) 'AIDS and Self Organisation of IV Drug Users', *International Journal of the Addictions*, vol. 22, no. 3, pp. 201-19

(December 16 1987) 'Gay Sex Teaching Move is Lost', *The Times*

Gifford-Jones, W. (October 27 1987) 'Mail on AIDS Victims shows Strongest Response is Fear', *Globe and Mail*, Toronto

Gilmore, Norbert (1988) 'Patient Care for AIDS', *Transplantation/Implantation Today*, vol. 5, Sept. pp. 47-50, Nov. pp. 27-30

_____ (1988) 'Sex, AIDS and Cultural Change', *The Sex Information and Education Council of Canada Journal*, vol. 3, no. 4, pp. 3-13

Ginzberg, Harold M., J. French, J. Jackson, P. I. Hartsock, M. G. MacDonald and S. H. Weiss (1986) 'Health Education and Knowledge Assessment of HTLV-III Diseases among Intravenous Drug Users', *Health Education Quarterly*, vol. 13, no. 4., pp. 373-82

Gostin, Larry and William J. Curran (1987) 'AIDS Screening, Confidentiality, and the Duty to Warn', *American Journal of Public Health*, vol. 77, no. 3, pp. 361-5

Green, John and David Miller (1986) *AIDS: The Story of a Disease,* London, Grafton Books

Hanlon, John J. and George E. Pickett (1984) *Public Health: Administration and Practice*, (8th edition) St Louis, Mosby

Hart, H. L. A. and A. M. Honoree (1959) *Causation in the Law*, Oxford, Clarendon Press

Hastings, G. B., D. S. Leather and A. C. Scott (1987) 'AIDS Publicity: Some Experiences from Scotland', *British Medical Journal*, vol. 294, no. 6563, pp. 48-9

Heyward, William L. and James W. Curran (1988) 'The Epidemiology of AIDS in the US', *Scientific American*, vol. 259, no. 4, pp. 72-81

Illingworth, Patricia (1988) 'The Friendship Model of Physician/Patient Relationship and Patient Autonomy', *Bioethics*, vol. 2, no.1, pp. 22-36

Kaplan, Howard B. (1975) *Self-Attitudes and Deviant Behavior*, Pacific Palisades, Calif., Goodyear Publishing Company

Kaplan, John (1988) 'Taking Drugs Seriously', *The Public Interest*, vol. 92, pp. 32-50

Kelly, Jeffrey A., J. S. St. Lawrence, S. Smith, H. V. Hood and D. J. Cook (1987) 'Medical Students' Attitudes Toward AIDS and Homosexual Patients', *Journal of Medical Education*, vol. 62, no. 7, pp. 549-56

Koehn, Hank E. (August 14 1987) 'My Passage Through AIDS', *Los Angeles Times*

Koop, C. Everett (1986) 'Surgeon General's Report on Acquired Immune Deficiency Syndrome', *Journal of the American Medical Association*, vol. 256, no. 20, pp. 2784-9

(February 3 1988) 'Lords Keep "Gay Clause" in Bill', *The Times*

(1988) *Lancet*, vol. 2, pp. 943-4

Macklin, Ruth (1986) 'Predicting Dangerousness and the Public Health Response to AIDS', *Hastings Center Report*, vol. 16, no. 6, pp. 16-23

Mann, Jonathan M., J. Chin, P. Piot and T. Quinn (1988) 'The International Epidemiology of AIDS', *Scientific American*, vol. 259, no. 4, pp. 82-9

Mayo, David J. (1988) 'AIDS Quarantines and Non-compliant Positives', in *AIDS: Ethics and Public Policy*, C. Pierce and D. VanDeVeer, eds, Belmont, Calif., Wadsworth Publishing Co., pp. 113-23

McGill Centre for Medicine, Ethics and Law (1988) *International Statistics*, prepared for the Symposium on the Economic Impact of HIV Infection

McKusick, Leon, W. Horstman and T. J. Coates (1985) 'AIDS and Sexual Behavior Reported by Gay Men in San Francisco', *American Journal of Public Health*, vol. 75, no. 5, pp. 493-6

McKusick, Leon, J. A. Wiley, T. J. Coates, R. Stall, G. Saika, S. Morin, K. Charles, W. Horstman and M. A. Conant (1985) 'Reported Changes in the Sexual Behavior of Men at Risk for AIDS, San Francisco, 1982-84 - The AIDS Behavioral Research Project', *Public Health Reports*, vol. 100, no. 6, pp. 622-9

McMearn, James H. (1972) 'Radical and Racial Perspectives on the Heroin Problem', in *"It's So Good Don't Even Try It Once": Heroin in Perspective*, D. E. Smith and G. R. Gay, eds, New Jersey, Prentice-Hall

Mill, John Stuart (1978) *John Stuart Mill: On Liberty*, E. Rapaport, ed., (Introduction by E. Rapaport), Indianapolis, Hackett Publishing Co.

_____ (1957) *Utilitarianism*, Oskar Piest, ed., Indianapolis, Bobbs-Merrill

Bibliographical References

Mohr, Richard D. (1987) 'AIDS, Gays and State Coercion', *Bioethics*, vol. 1, no. 1, pp. 35-50

_____ (forthcoming) *Gays/Justice: A Study of Ethics, Society and Law*, New York, Columbia University Press

Nadelmann, Ethan A. (1988) 'The Case for Legalization', *The Public Interest*, vol. 92, pp. 3-31

Nickel, James W. (1977) 'Classification by Race in Compensatory Programs', *Philosophical Issues in Law: Cases and Materials*, Kenneth Kipnis, ed., New Jersey, Prentice-Hall, pp. 235-40

O'Farrell, Elaine (September 8 1987) 'Canadians Still Harbor Myths and Many Fears About AIDS', *Medical Post*

Pierce, Christine and Donald VanDeVeer (1988) *AIDS: Ethics and Public Policy*, Belmont, Calif., Wadsworth Publishing Co.

Preston, John, ed., (1985) *Hot Living: Erotic Stories About Safe Sex*, Boston, Alyson Publications

Rawls, John (1971) *A Theory of Justice*, Cambridge, Harvard University Press

Raz, Joseph (1986) *The Morality of Freedom*, Oxford, Clarendon Press

Rechy, John (1977) *The Sexual Outlaw*, New York, Grove Press

Regush, Nicholas (May 22 1988) 'The Kidney Patients Britain Allows to Die', *Montreal Gazette*

Rutherford, George (forthcoming) 'HIV Infection: Outcome and Survival', *Proceedings of International Symposium on the Economic Impact of HIV Infection in Canada*, Montreal, McGill Centre for Medicine, Ethics and Law

Shilts, Randy (1987) *And The Band Played On: Politics, People, and the AIDS Epidemic*, New York, St Martin's Press

Somerville, Margaret and Norbert Gilmore (1988) *Human Immunodeficiency Virus Antibody Testing*, Montreal, McGill Centre for Medicine, Ethics and Law

Titmuss, Richard M. (1972) *The Gift Relationship: From Human Blood to Social Policy*, New York, Vintage Books

Wasserstrom, Richard (1978) 'A Defense of Programs of Preferential Treatment', *National Forum*, vol. 58, no. 1, pp. 15-18

Watlington, Dennis (1987) 'Between the Cracks', *Vanity Fair*, vol. 50, no. 12, pp. 146-51, pp. 184-6

Weinberg, Martin S. and Colin J. Williams (1974) *Male Homosexuals: Their Problems and Adaptations*, New York, Oxford University Press

_____ (1975) 'Gay Bathhouses and the Social Organisation of Impersonal Sex', *Social Problems*, vol. 23, no. 2, pp. 124-36

Wikler, Daniel I. (1978) 'Persuasion and Coercion for Health: Ethical Issues in Government Efforts to Change Life-styles', *Milbank Memorial Fund Quarterly/Health and Society*, vol. 56, no. 3, pp. 303-38

Young, Robert (1980) 'Autonomy and the Inner Self', *American Philosophical Quarterly*, vol. 17, no. 1, pp. 35-43

Bibliography

Acheson, E. D. (March 22 1986) 'AIDS: A Challenge for the Public Health', *The Lancet*, vol. 1, no. 8482, pp. 662-6

(January 17 1988) 'AIDS Antibodies in New York Infants', *New York Times*

(October 10 1987) 'AIDS in the U. K.', *The Lancet*, vol. 2, no. 8563, p. 869

(February 4 1988) 'AIDS Sufferers Need Reassurance', *The Times*

Arrow, K. J. (1973) *Individual Choice Under Certainty and Uncertainty*, Cambridge, Belknap Press

_____ (1986) *Social Choice and Justice*, London, Basil Blackwell

Bakalar, J. B. and L. Grinspoon (1984) *Drug Control in a Free Society*, Cambridge, Cambridge University Press

_____ (1984) 'Drug Abuse Policy and Social Attitudes to Risk-Taking', in *Feeling Good and Doing Better: Ethics and Nontherapeutic Drug Use*, T. M. Murray, W. Gaylin and R. Macklin (eds), New Jersey, Humana Press Inc., pp. 13-26

Barber, John (June 15 1987) 'Confrontation and Concern about AIDS', *Maclean's*, pp. 40-1

Beauchamp, Dan E. (1975) 'The Alcohol Alibi: Blaming Alcoholics', *Society*, vol. 12, pp. 12-17

_____ (1975) 'Public Health: Alien Ethic In A Strange Land', *American Journal of Public Health*, vol. 65, no. 12, pp. 1338-9

Beecham, Linda (1987) 'Further Legal Opinion on HIV Testing Being Sought', *British Medical Journal*, vol. 295, no. 6612, p. 1577

Berzon, B. and R. Leighton (eds), (1979) *Positively Gay: New Approaches in Gay Life*, Millbrae, Calif., Celestial Arts

Bishop, Anne H. and J. R. Scudder (1987) 'Nursing Ethics in an Age of Controversy', *Advanced Nursing Science*, vol. 9, no. 3, pp. 34-43

Bloom, David E. and Geoffrey Carliner (1988) 'The Economic Impact of AIDS in the United States', *Science*, vol. 239, pp. 604-9

Bok, Sissela (1982) *Secrets: On the Ethics of Concealment and Revelation*, New York, Pantheon Books

Boswell, J. (1980) *Christianity, Social Tolerance and Homosexuality: Gay People in Western Europe From the Beginning of the Christian Era to the Fourteenth Century*, Chicago, University of Chicago Press

Brandt, Allan M. (1985) *No Magic Bullet: A Social History of Venereal Disease in the United States Since 1880*, New York, Oxford University Press

Breckenridge, Joan (March 1 1988) 'Canada's First AIDS Hospice', *Globe and Mail, Toronto*

Brigham, David P. (1986) 'You Never Told Me ... You Never Asked; Tort Liability for the Sexual Transmission of Aids', *Dickinson Law Review*, vol. 91, pp. 529-52

Buchanan, Allen E. (1984) 'The Right to a Decent Minimum of Health Care', *Philosophy and Public Affairs*, vol. 13, pp. 55-78

Buckley, William F. (March 18 1986) 'Identify All the Carriers', *New York Times*

Burke, Donald S., J. F. Brundage, J. R. Herbold, W. Berner, L. I. Gardner, J. D. Gunzenhauser, J. Voskovitch and R. R. Redfield (1987) 'Human Immunodeficiency Virus Infections Among Civilian Applicants For United States Military Service, October 1985 to March 1986: Demographic Factors Associated With Seropositivity', *New England Journal of Medicine*, vol. 317, no. 3, pp. 131-6

Calabrese, Leonard H., B. Harris, K. A. Easley and M. R. Proffitt (1986) 'Persistence of High Risk Sexual Activity Among Homosexual Men in an Area of Low Incidence for Acquired Immunodeficiency Syndrome', *AIDS Research*, vol. 2, no. 4, pp. 357-61

(December 2 1987) 'Californians will Again Vote on Isolating Victims of AIDS', *New York Times*

Campbell, M. J. and W. E. Waters (1987) 'Public Knowledge about AIDS Increasing', *British Medical Journal*, vol. 294, no. 6576, p. 892-3

Campbell, R. (1979) *Self-love and Self-respect: A Philosphical Study of Egoism*, Ottawa, Canadian Library of Philosophy

Cassens, Brett J. (1985) 'Social Consequences of the Acquired Immunodeficiency Syndrome', *Annals of Internal Medicine*, vol. 103, no. 5, pp. 768-71

Cecchi, Robert L. (1986) 'Health Advocacy for AIDS Patients', *Quality Review Bulletin*, vol. 12, no. 8, pp. 297-303

Check, William (1985) 'Public Education on AIDS: Not Only the Media's Responsibility', *Hastings Center Report*, vol. 15, no. 4, pp. 27-31

Bibliographical References

Coates, Thomas J., L. Temoshok and J. Mandel (1984) 'Psychosocial Research Is Essential to Understanding and Treating AIDS', *American Psychologist*, vol. 39, p. 1309-14

Conrad, John P. (1984) 'Controlling the Uncontrollable', in *Feeling Good and Doing Better: Ethics and Nontherapeutic Drug Use*, T. M. Murray, W. Gaylin and R. Macklin (eds), New Jersey, Humana Press Inc., pp. 49-64

Crossette, Barbara (November 8 1987) 'Fear of AIDS Surfaces in Permissive Bangkok', *New York Times*

Curran, James W., H. W. Jaffe, A. M. Hardy, W. M. Morgan, R. M. Selik and T. J. Dondero (1988) 'Epidemiology of HIV Infection and AIDS in the United States', *Science*, vol. 239, pp. 610-16

Daniels, Norman (1985) *Just Health Care*, Cambridge, Cambridge University Press

DeCecco, John P., ed. (1984) *Homophobia: An Overview*, New York, Howorth Press

D'Emilio, John (1983) *Sexual Politics, Sexual Communities: The Making of a Homosexual Minority in the United States, 1940-1970*, Chicago, University of Chicago Press

Dickens, Bernard M. (1988) 'Legal Rights and Duties in the AIDS Epidemic', *Science*, vol. 239, pp. 580-6

Dilsaver, S. C. and Jeffrey A. Coffman (1987) 'Effect of Generous Funding for AIDS Research on General Biomedical Research', *New England Journal of Medicine*, vol. 318, no. 16, pp. 1071-2

Doherty, John P. (1986) 'AIDS: One Psychosocial Response', *Quality Review Bulletin*, vol. 12, no. 8, pp. 295-7

(June 20 1987) 'Drug Addicts With Dirty Needles', *The Nation*

Dworkin, Ronald (1977) *Taking Rights Seriously*, Cambridge, Mass., Harvard University Press

Edwards, W. and A. Tversky (1967) *Decision Making: Selected Readings*, Harmondsworth, Penguin

Elster, Jon (1985) 'Weakness of Will and the Free-Rider Problem', *Economics and Philosophy*, vol. 1, pp. 231-65

———— ed. (1986) *Rational Choice*, New York, New York University Press

———— (1979) *Ulysses and the Sirens: Studies in Rationality and Irrationality*, New York, Cambridge University Press

Elster, Jon and A. Hylland (eds), (1986) *Foundations of Social Choice Theory*, Cambridge, Cambridge University Press

Feinberg, Joel (1984) *Offense to Others*, Oxford, Oxford University Press

Ferrara, Anthony J. (1984) 'My Personal Experience With AIDS', *American Psychologist*, vol. 39, no. 11, pp. 1285-7

(January 13 1988) 'Fire Brigade Ignore Call to Help Baby with AIDS', *Montreal Gazette*

(January 26 1988) 'Firing Unfair Says Nurse with AIDS', *Montreal Gazette*

Fitzgerald, Frances (July 21 1986) 'A Reporter at Large -The Castro-I', *New Yorker*, pp. 34-70

Flam, Robin and Zena Stein (1986) 'Behaviour, Infection, and Immune Response: An Epidemiological Approach', in *The Social Dimensions of AIDS: Method and Theory*, D. A. Feldman and T. M. Johnson (eds), New York, Praeger, pp. 61-76

(January 1988) 'Florida Considering Locking up Some Carriers of the AIDS Virus', *New York Times*

Freedman, Benjamin (1988) 'Health Professions, Codes and the Right to Refuse to Treat HIV-Infectious Patients', *Hastings Center Report*, vol. 18, no. 2, pp. 20-5

French, Orland (March 3 1988) 'Coming out of the Closet to Crusade', *Globe and Mail, Toronto*

(December 18 1987) 'Gay Groups Condemn "Bigot's Charter"', *New Society*

(January 29 1988) 'Gays, AIDS and the Government', *New Society*

Geis, G., R. Wright, T. Garrett and P. R. Wilson (1976) 'Reported Consequences of Decriminalization of Consensual Adult Homosexuality in Seven American States', *Journal of Homosexuality*, vol. 1, no. 4, pp. 419-26

Gostin, Larry (1986) 'The Future of Communicable Disease Control: Toward a New Concept in Public Health Law', *The Milbank Quarterly*, vol. 64, Suppl. 1, pp. 79-117

Gostin, Larry and William J. Curran (1986) 'The Limits of Compulsion in Controlling AIDS', *Hastings Center Report*, vol. 16, no. 6, pp. 24-9

Gostin, Larry and Andrew Ziegler (1987) 'A Review of AIDS-Related Legislative and Regulatory Policy in the United States', *Law, Medicine, and Health*, vol. 15, nos 1-2, pp. 5-16

Bibliographical References

Gunn, Sheila (February 2 1988) 'Gay Ban Clause Approved', *The Times*
_____ (February 4 1988) 'Government Stays Adamant on "Homosexuals Clause", *The Times*
_____ (January 26 1988) 'Peers May Alter Gay Clause', *The Times*
Guttmacher, Sally (1971) 'Whole in Body, Mind and Spirit: Holistic Health and the Limits of Medicine', *Hastings Center Report*, vol. 9, no. 2, pp. 15-21
Hammond, J. D. and Arnold F. Shapiro (1986) 'AIDS and the Limits of Insurability', *The Milbank Quarterly*, vol. 64, Suppl. 1, pp. 143-67
(March 8 1988) 'HIV Infection is not Spreading into Heterosexuals in London', *Medical Post*
(January 19 1988) 'HIV is No Risk in Families', *Medical Post*
Holmes, William (February 19 1988) 'Courage in Face of AIDS', *The Times*
Hughes, Colin (December 9 1987) 'Move to Ban Gay Teaching is Backed by Labour', *Independent*
(January 26 1988) 'Illinois Health System is Taxed by Law Requiring Pre-nuptial AIDS Tests', *New York Times*
Johnston, Cameron (January 5 1988) 'Doctors Stereotyping AIDS Patients, Often Unwittingly', *Medical Post*
_____ (December 22 1987) 'Fee for Anonymous AIDS Test under Proposed Law', *Medical Post*
Jones, R. W. and J. E. Bates (1978) 'Satisfaction in Male Homosexual Couples', *Journal of Homosexuality*, vol. 3, no. 3, pp. 217-24
Josephson, Eric and Eleanor E. Carroll (1974) *Drug Use: Epidemiological and Sociological Approaches*, Washington, Hemisphere Publishing
Judson, Horace F. (1974) *Heroin Addiction in Britain; What Americans Can Learn from the English Experience*, New York, Harcourt Brace Jovanovich
Kahn, Alfred E. (1966) 'The Tyranny of Small Decisions: Market Failures, Imperfections, and the Limits of Economics', *Kyklos*, vol. 19, no. 1, pp. 23-47
Kaplan, John (1987) 'Stigmatization of AIDS Patients by Physicians', *American Journal of Public Health*, vol. 77, no. 1, pp. 789-91
Kerr, Peter (February 1 1988) 'Weighing of 2 Perils Led to Needles-for-Addicts Plan', *New York Times*
Kingman, Sharon (1988) 'AIDS and the Social Outcast', *New Scientist*, vol. 10, pp. 30-1

Kirby, M. D. (1986) 'AIDS Legislation - Turning up the Heat?', *Journal of Medical Ethics*, vol. 12, no. 14, pp. 107-13

Kotarba, Joseph A. and Norris G. Lang (1986) 'Gay Lifestyle Change and AIDS: Preventative Health Care', in *The Social Dimensions of AIDS: Method and Theory*, D. A. Feldman and T. M. Johnson (eds), New York, Praeger, pp. 127-43

Krim, Mathilde (1985) 'AIDS: The Challenge to Science and Medicine', *Hastings Center Report*, vol. 15, no. 4, pp. 2-7

Kristof, Nicholas D. (June 17 1987) 'Hong Kong Program: Addicts Without AIDS', *New York Times*

Lalani, Shamin (1986) 'The Plague of Panic', *Canadian Doctor*

Lappé, Mark (1982) 'Values and Public Health: Value Considerations in Setting Health Policy', *Theoretical Medicine*, no. 4, pp. 71-92

Lauritsen, John (October 19 1987) 'AZT on Trial', *New York Native*

Levine, Carol (1986) 'AIDS: Public Health and Civil Liberties', *Hastings Center Report*, vol. 16, no. 6, pp. 1-2

_____ (1986) 'AIDS: An Ethical Challenge for Our Time', *Quality Review Bulletin*, vol. 12, no. 8, pp. 273-7

Levine, Carol and Ronald Bayer (1985) 'Screening Blood: Public Health and Medical Uncertainty', *Hastings Center Report*, vol. 15, no. 4, pp. 8-11

Lieberson, J., M. F. Silverman, M. Krim, R. Bayer, G. Friedland, G. MacDonald, A. Giudici Fettner, S. Schultz, A. M. Brandt and M. J. Shebar (1986) 'AIDS: What is to be Done?', *Harper's Magazine*, vol. 271, no. 1625, pp. 39-52

Lohr, Steve (February 29 1988) 'There's No Preaching just the Clean Needles', *New York Times*

Longley, Clifford (December 29 1987) 'Bishops to Ban Gays in Clergy', *The Times*

MacArthur, Brian (January 31 1988) 'When Private Action becomes Public Property', *The Sunday Times*

Macklin, R. and G. Friedland (1986) 'AIDS Research: The Ethics of Clinical Trials', *Law, Medicine and Health Care*, vol. 14, nos 5-6, pp. 273-80

Marotta, Toby (1981) *The Politics of Homosexuality*, Boston, Houghton Mifflin

Bibliographical References

Martin, Jeannee P. (1986) 'Ensuring Quality Hospice Care for the Person with AIDS', *Quality Review Bulletin*, vol. 12, no. 10, pp. 353-8

Martin, John L. (1986) 'AIDS Risk Reduction Recommendations and Sexual Behavior Patterns among Gay Men: A Multifactorial Categorial Approach to Assessing Change', *Health Education Quarterly*, vol. 13, no. 4, pp. 347-58

_____ (1987) 'The Impact of AIDS on Gay Male Sexual Behavior Patterns in New York City', *American Journal of Public Health*, vol. 77, no. 5, pp. 578-81

McCombie, S. C. (1986) 'The Cultural Impact of the "AIDS" Test: The American Experience', *Social Science and Medicine*, vol. 23, no. 5, pp. 455-9

McCormick, Ann, H. Tillett, B. Bannister and J. Emslie (1987) 'Surveillance of AIDS in the United Kingdom', *British Medical Journal*, vol. 295, no. 6611, pp. 1466-9

McGavran, Edward G. (1953) 'What is Public Health?', *Canadian Journal of Public Health*, vol. 44, no. 12, pp. 441-51

McGuirl, Marlene and Robert N. Gee (1985) 'AIDS: An Overview of the British, Australian, and American Responses', *Hofstra Law Review*, vol. 14, pp. 107-35

(July 22 1986) 'MDs Urged: Test Patients for HTLV Antibodies Only After Getting their Informed Consent', *Canadian Family Physician*, vol. 32, pp. 1423-5

Merritt, Deborah J. (1986) 'The Constitutional Balance Between Health and Liberty', *Hastings Center Report*, vol. 16, no. 6, pp. 2-10

Michael, Lewis and Jeanne Brooks-Gunn (1979) *Social Cognition and the Acquisition of Self*, New York, Plenum Press

Milio, Nancy (1976) 'A Framework for Prevention: Changing Health-Damaging to Health-Generating Life Patterns', *American Journal of Public Health*, vol. 66, no. 5, pp. 435-9

Mills, Michael, C. B. Wofsy and J. Mills (1986) 'The Acquired Immunodeficiency Syndrome', *New England Journal of Medicine*, vol. 314, no. 14, pp. 931-6

Minor, James R. (1987) 'Current Treatment Approaches', *American Pharmacy*, vol. NS27, no. 8, pp. 36-42

Montefiore, Alan, ed. (1979) *Philosophy and Personal Relations; An Anglo-French Study*, Montreal, McGill-Queen's University Press

Morgan, Thomas (February 5 1988) 'Inside a "Shooting Gallery": New Front in the AIDS War', *New York Times*

Morin, Stephen F., K. A. Charles and A. K. Malyon (1984) 'The Psychological Impact of AIDS on Gay Men', *American Psychologist*, vol. 39, no. 11, pp. 1288-93

Moser, Robert H. (1986) 'Introduction', *Quality Review Bulletin*, vol. 12, no. 8, pp. 270-2

Murray, Terry (March 8 1988) 'No Hetero AIDS Epidemic', *Medical Post*

Musto, David F. (1973) *The American Disease: Origins of Narcotics Control*, New Haven, Yale University Press

_____ (1986) 'Quarantine and the Problem of AIDS', *The Milbank Quarterly*, vol. 64, Suppl. 1, pp. 97-117

Nau, Jean-Yves and Frank Nouchi (February 21 1988) 'Call for Routine Testing for AIDS', *Manchester Guardian Weekly*, vol. 138, no. 8, pp. 14

(August 4 1986) 'Needling AIDS', *Time*

Nelson, M. C. and J. Ikenberry (eds), (1979) *Psychosexual Imperatives: Their Role in Identity Formation*, New York, Human Sciences Press

Neville, Robert (1984) 'The State's Intervention in Individuals' Drug Use', in *Feeling Good and Doing Better: Ethics and Nontherapeutic Drug Use*, T. M. Murray, W. Gaylin and R. Macklin (eds), New Jersey, Humana Press Inc., pp. 65-80

Newman, Robert G. (1987) 'Methadone Treatment', *New England Journal of Medicine*, vol. 317, no. 7, pp. 447-50

(January 29 1988) 'No Need for Free Syringes or Explicit Ads in AIDS Battle: Epp', *Montreal Gazette*

(January 13 1988) 'N.S. Health Minister Wants to Isolate AIDS Carriers', *Montreal Gazette*

Ostrow, David G. and Gayle C. Terence (1986) 'Psychosocial and Ethical Issues of AIDS Health Care Programs', *Quality Review Bulletin*, vol. 12, no. 10, pp. 292-4

Panem, Sandra (1985) 'AIDS: Public Policy and Biomedical Research', *Hastings Center Report*, vol. 15, no. 4, pp. 23-6

Parmet, Wendy E. (1985) 'AIDS and Quarantine: The Revival of an Archaic Doctrine', *Hofstra Law Review*, vol. 14, pp. 53-90

(February 2 1988) 'Peers Throw out Amendment to "Gay Clause"', *The Times*

Bibliographical References

Plummer, Kenneth (1975) *Sexual Stigma: An Interactionist Account*, London, Routledge and Kegan Paul

Prentice, Thomas (February 9 1988) 'Women Face Increased Risk of Catching AIDS', *The Times*

_____ (February 19 1988) 'GPs Ignorant and Prejudiced about AIDS', *The Times*

(December 4 1987) 'Private School will Begin AIDS Testing', *Globe and Mail*, Toronto

(1986) 'Public Information Campaign on AIDS', *The Lancet*, vol. 1, no. 8482, p. 694

Quadland, Michael C. and William D. Shattls (1987) 'AIDS, Sexuality and Sexual Control', *Journal of Homosexuality*, vol. 3, no. 4, pp. 277-98

Rabin, Judith A. (1986) 'The AIDS Epidemic and Gay Bathhouses: A Constitutional Analysis', *Journal of Health Politics, Policy, and Law*, vol. 10, no. 4, pp. 729-47

(March 8 1988) 'Researchers Can't Prove Claim Heterosexual AIDS "Rampant"', *Montreal Gazette*

Richards, D. A. J. (1982) *Sex, Drugs, Death and the Law: An Essay on Human Rights and Overcriminalization*, New Jersey, Rowman and Littlefield

Roberts, Paul (1987) 'Sex and Death', *Toronto Life*

Robertson, Geoffrey (June 1 1988) 'Fear Not Clause 28, only the Prejudice Behind it', *Guardian*

Rubington, Earl and Martin S. Weinberg (eds), (1973) *Deviance, The Interactionist Perspective; Text and Readings in the Sociology of Deviance*, New York, Macmillan Publishing Co.

Sagaran, E. (1975) *Deviants and Deviance: An Introduction to the Study of Disvalued People and Behavior*, New York, Praeger Publishers

Schwartz, William A. (June 20 1987) 'Drug Addicts With Dirty Needles', *The Nation*, pp. 843-6

Scitovsky, Anne A. and D. P. Rice (1987) 'Estimates of the Direct and Indirect Costs of Acquired Immunodeficiency Syndrome in the United States, 1985, 1986, and 1991', *Public Health Reports*, vol. 102, no. 1, pp. 5-17

Silverman, Mervyn F. and Deborah B. Silverman (1985) 'AIDS and the Threat to Public Health', *Hastings Center Report*, vol. 15, no. 4, pp. 19-22

Sinclair, K. and M. W. Ross (1985) 'Consequences of Decriminalization of Homosexuality: A Study of Two Australian States', *Journal of Homosexuality*, vol. 12, no. 1

Smilgis, Martha (February 16 1987) 'The Big Chill: Fear of AIDS', *Time*

Somerville, Margaret (1980) *Consent to Medical Care*, Protection of Life Project, Law Reform Commission Of Canada

Stapleton, Dan (1986) 'AIDS: Psychosocial Dimensions', *Canadian Family Physician*, vol. 32, pp. 2510-17

Sullivan, Ronald (June 8 1986) 'Cost of AIDS Care is Half what was Projected, Economist Reports', *New York Times*

Szasz, Thomas S. (1987) 'AIDS and Drugs: Balancing Risks and Benefits', *The Lancet*, vol. 2, no. 8556, p. 450

Tehan, Claire B. (1986) 'Training Volunteers in Home Care for Patients with AIDS', *Quality Review Bulletin*, vol. 12, no. 10, pp. 359-60

Thomas, Owen (March 14-20 1988) 'Ex-gays Direct Others to a Road out of Homosexuality', *Christian Science Monitor*, p. 8

Tuller, N. R. (1978) 'Couples: The Hidden Segment of the Gay World', *Journal of Homosexuality*, vol. 3, no. 4, pp. 331-43

(November 27 1987) 'U.K. Compensation for AIDS Haemophiliacs', *Scrip*, no. 1261

Veatch, Robert M. (1983) 'Voluntary Risks to Health: The Ethical Issues', in *Moral Problems in Medicine*, R. Macklin and S. Gorovitz (eds), New Jersey, Prentice-Hall

_____ (1974) 'Who Should Pay for Smokers' Health Care?', *Hastings Center Report*, vol. 4, no. 5, pp. 8-9

Volberding, Paul and Donald Abrams (1985) 'Clinical Care and Research in AIDS', *Hastings Center Report*, vol. 15, no. 4, pp. 16-23

Walker, Lou Ann (June 21 1987) 'What Comforts AIDS Families', *New York Times Magazine*, pp. 16-22, 63, 78

Walters, LeRoy (1988) 'Ethical Issues in the Prevention and Treatment of HIV Infection and AIDS', *Science*, vol. 239, pp. 597-603

Weeks, J. (1979) *Coming Out: Homosexual Politics in Britain, from the Nineteenth Century to the Present*, London, Quartet Books

Wells, Nicholas (1986) *The AIDS Virus: Forecasting its Impact*, London, Office of Health Economics

Wicklund, Robert A. (1974) *Freedom and Reactance*, New York, John Wiley and Sons

Bibliographical References

Wilkerson, Isabel (January 26 1988) 'Prenuptial AIDS Screening a Strain in Illinois', *New York Times*

Winkelstein, Warren Jr., M. Samuel, N. S. Padian, J. A. Wiley, W. Lang, R. E. Anderson and J. A. Levy (1987) 'The San Francisco Men's Health Study: III. Reduction in Human Immunodeficiency Virus Transmission among Homosexual/Bisexual Men 1982-86', *American Journal of Public Health*, vol. 76, no. 9, pp. 685-9

Zuckerman, Arie J. (1986) 'Would Screening Prevent the International Spread of AIDS?', *The Lancet*, vol. 2, no. 8517, pp. 1208-9

ability-based health care 154-6
adaptive desires 119
adaptive preference 63-4, 74, 79, 92-3, 97n2, 101n55, 116, 122, 167
affirmative action 141, 159
AIDS awareness programs 83, 130-1
alternative therapies 9, 83, 157
altruism 135n21
anal receptive intercourse 7, 37, 58n23, 67-8, 98nn14,16
Anderson, Digby 129
Anne, Princess 120
anti-paternalism 56n3
antibody status 41-4, 46, 58n20, 59n35, 107-8. *See also* duty to disclose
antiviral drugs 9
"anyone who would do that" argument 69-72
acquired immunodeficiency syndrome. *See* HIV/AIDS
autonomy
    autonomous desires 161-3; behavior change 164-5, 173n36; celebration of 13; coercion and manipulation 74-83; compensation 156-8; definition of 62-3, 97n3; disadvantaged minorities 91-3; enhancement of 65, 158, 162-4, 173n32; health care 151-6; high-risk behavior 14, 23-4, 63, 67-9, 73, 97n2, 99n21; HIV/AIDS education 162-8, 173n36; human capacity for 10-11, 17, 168; ignorance 83-90; obstacles to 23, 67, 73, 98n13, 105, 133; options 11, 64-5, 93, 103, 156; psychoanalysis 173n32; psychotherapy 65; self-inflicted harm 25; voluntary

action 36-7; weak harm principle 114-16. *See also* legislation and social policy
azidothymidine 8-9
AZT. *See* azidothymidine

Bartky, Sandra 65
Bassford, Skip 57n15
Bayer, Ronald 46, 49-52
Beauchamp, Dan E. 46, 48-9
Bell, Alan P. 75, 94
Black, David 77
Blacks 1, 65, 91-3, 119, 141-2, 159, 171n8
"blame the victim" argument 93-6, 120
Blendon, Robert J. 111
blood transfusion recipients 7
BMW-desire 116-17, 119 *See also* yuppie-desires
bonding mechanism and needle-sharing 101n56
Bowers v. Hardwick 129
Britain 23, 28, 93, 128-29, 151-2, 172n21
British Kidney Patients Association 151-2
British National Health Service 152
Bursztajn, Harold 57n14

Callahan, Daniel 171n16
Canada 6, 110-11, 152, 172n21
Castro District 85, 100n41
causal responsibility 29-30, 37-40
CDC. *See* Centers for Disease Control
Centers for Disease Control 4, 5, 68
chronic lymphadenopathy 5
Clause 28 128-9

Index

coercion 56n3, 67, 73-4, 78-80, 98n13
cognitive dissonance 64, 97n6
collective harms 46-7
collectivized health care systems 152, 172n21
compensation
    criterion of eligibility for 158-9; distribution of 159-61; health care 16-17, 144-58, 172nn19,22,27; justice-based 141; and the law 170n6, 171n8; Mohr's argument 144-9, 155; monetary 17, 138, 158-61; practical considerations of 158-61; preferential hiring 141-2; compensatory justice 141-3
competency 69-73, 99nn18,22
condom use 39, 58n23, 59n32, 68.
    See also safe sex (safer sex).
consent to harm 27-8
consequentialism 31, 42, 57n13
contract-tracing 133
criterion of foreseeability 38-9, 58nn28,29
Curran, James W. 19n9, 68
Curran, William J. 106-9

decriminalization of homosexual sodomy 129
decriminalization of narcotic use 95, 101n56
depression 43, 59n36
desert-based health care 153-4
disadvantaged minorities 91-3
discrimination
    against Blacks 93, 141-2, 159; against gay men 15-18, 77-8, 121, 127-32, 142, 143-4, 156, 166-7; against Hispanics 93, 141 against IV drug-users 15-18, 95-6, 142, 143-4, 170n5; against

persons with HIV/AIDS 131-2; against women 141-2, 154; discriminatory attitudes of health professionals 131-2; discriminatory laws against gay men 78, 121, 128-30, 136n38; positive discrimination 141
Donelan, Karen 111
Dreuilhe, Emmanuel 4, 59n36, 111
drug therapies 8-9
Duckett, Margaret 98n16
duty to disclose HIV/AIDS status 31-6, 40-4, 58n20, 59n35
Dworkin, Gerald 62-3, 97n3

efficiency-based arguments 105-13
Elster, Jon 97n6
epidemiology of HIV/AIDS 1-2, 6-8, 20n19, 68, 91
equal opportunity 113, 121-2, 126, 127

family life of gay men 145-8, 171n12
fast track. *See under* gay men
fear of HIV/AIDS 2, 3, 105, 109-12, 131, 133
fear used in HIV/AIDS educational programs 101n45, 164-8
Feinberg, Joel 27
Fineberg, Harvey V. 164
Finn, Peter 128
Fitzgerald, Frances 84
Frankfurt, Harry 97n3, 99n20
Freedman, Benjamin 99n19
freedom, negative and positive 18
free riding 139

Gallo, Robert 6
gay clause. *See* Clause 28

gay community 41-3, 59n36, 68, 77, 84-9, 90, 95, 100n41, 127, 164
gay men
    bathhouses 14, 70, 84, 86-9, 94, 113; Bowers v. Hardwick 129; causal responsibility of 37-40; compensation for 158-61; consent to harm 27; duty to disclose HIV/AIDS status 31-4, 40-4, 59n35; discrimination against 15-18, 77-8, 127-32, 136n38, 142, 143-4, 156, 166-7; discriminatory laws against 78, 121, 128-30, 136n38; family life of 145-8, 171n12; fast track 44, 59n30, 63, 77-9, 98n15, 117, 119, 122, 140, 148; gay liberation 98n15, 130; high-risk behavior of 7-8, 14, 24, 31-2, 36-46, 58nn23,29, 67-8, 70-1, 74-9, 83-9, 93-6, 97n2, 98nn15,16, 99nn21,23,24, 113, 137, 140; HIV/AIDS education for 50, 83-9, 101n45, 138, 162-8; marriage of 95; moral responsibility of 40-6; self-esteem of 16, 125-7; self-inflicted harm 36-7 social attitudes about 75, 94; social harms against 94-5, 117-20, 133 143-4, 168-9; socially induced desires of 117-20; stereotyping of 77-8; subculture 78; as thrill seekers 86; transmission of HIV/AIDS 7-8, 36-7, 42, 44-5, 46, 68, 84
Gifford-Jones, W. 110
Gilmore, Norbert 98n16, 99n21, 164-5
good life 66, 122
good society 10-18, 23-4, 56n3, 61, 103-4, 113, 115-16, 122, 124-5, 126, 133, 142, 161, 163, 168.
Gostin, Larry 106
government interference 10-12, 15. *See also* legislation and social policy

harm principle 24-6, 37, 56n3, 61-2, 66, 93, 104, 113-16, 124, 133
harm to others 11, 24-6, 36, 45-6, 103
harm to self 11, 24, 27, 33, 36-7, 40, 45-6, 58n21, 104
health care
    ability-based 154-8; as compensation 16-17, 144-57, 172nn19,22,27; economic costs of 151-2, 171n16; Mohr's argument for state-funded 144-9; need-based 151-4; preferential health care 152-3, 172n19; voucher system 157
Herpes zoster infection 7
heterosexuals 28, 58n24, 63, 78, 83, 94, 95, 97n5, 99n24, 121
Heyward, William L. 19n9, 68
high-risk behavior. *See under* gay men *and* IV drug-users
Hispanics 1-2, 91-3, 142
HIV/AIDS
    AIDS virus 6; lifestyle disease 139-40; awareness programs 83, 130-1; Blacks in US 91; Brazil 6; Canada 6; diagnosis of 6-7; discrimination against persons with 131-2; duty to disclose status of 31-6, 40-4, 58n20, 59n35; economic and social costs of 53-5; education 50, 83-90, 101n45, 138, 162-8; epidemiology of 1-2, 6; Europe 6; fear of 2-3, 105, 109-12, 131, 133; France 6; health care as

compensation 16-17, 144-58, 172nn19,22,27; Hispanics in US 91; Italy 6; leukaemia patients 131-2; mandatory testing 11, 22, 106-9; moral and social challenge of 9-18; accounts of persons with 2-4; press coverage of 83; public health 46-52; public opinion about 110-13; San Francisco 84-6; transmission of 7-8, 28-9, 38-9, 42, 44-6, 50, 68, 103-4; treatment of persons with 8-9; United Kingdom 6; United States 4-6, 91; vaccine for 9, 107, 109. *See also* legislation and social policy

homophobia 127. *See also* discrimination

homosexuals. *See* gay men

hospice care 144-5, 147-51, 155. *See also* health care

HTLV-III 46, 49-51

human immunodeficiency virus. *See* HIV/AIDS

ignorance 67, 73, 83, 90, 98n13

impersonal sex 38, 40-1, 44, 58n23, 59n33, 68-9, 70-1, 75-8, 94-5, 99n24, 166-7. *See also* multiple anonymous sex

incompetency 67, 69-73, 98n13, 99n23

independent agents 97n2

injection equipment 24, 28, 72, 81-2, 90, 91, 93, 100n33, 101n56, 140

interferon 9

intravenous drug-users. *See* IV drug-users

IV drug-users
causal responsibility 29-30; compensation for 158-61; consent to harm 27-8; discrimination against 15-18, 93, 96, 142-4, 170n5; duty to disclose HIV/AIDS status 31-6; friendships of 34-6; "giving them their wings" 80; high-risk behavior of 7-8, 24, 28-36, 40, 61-4, 67-8, 72-4, 79-83, 89-96, 99nn21,23, 104, 113, 137, 140, 142; HIV/AIDS education for 89-90, 138, 162-4; injection equipment 24, 28, 72, 81-2, 90, 91, 93, 100n33, 140; involuntary withdrawal 81-2; moral responsibility 30-6, 57n13; needle-sharing 28-31, 90, 100n33, 118; running partners 80-1; self-esteem of 92, 125-7; self-inflicted harm 28-9, 36, 58n21; shooting galleries 80-2, 140; social harms against 95-6, 117-20, 123-4, 133, 143-4, 168-9; socially induced desires of 118-20; sterilized equipment 101n56; subculture 92-3, 101n56; transmission of HIV/AIDS 7-8, 28, 49-51

Kaposi's sarcoma 5, 7, 8, 85

Koop, C. Everett 46

KS. *See* Kaposi's sarcoma

legislation and social policy 2, 9, 11, 13-18, 23-5, 49, 52, 53-5, 66-7, 97n1, 103-5, 108-9, 114-16, 122-4, 133, 135n21, 136n38, 137-8, 141-3, 168-9, 170n6, 171n16; Belgium 22; Britain 23, 128-9;

Costa Rica 22; France 22-3; Germany 22; Italy 23; Netherlands 23; United States 53, 129-30, 142, 154-6, 159
liberalism 10, 18. *See also* Mill, John Stuart
liberty 9-13, 65-7, 112-13, 127, 132-3, 168; negative and positive freedom 18
life-plans 10, 12, 121-2, 124-7, 168
lifestyle argument 139-41
lifestyle disease 139-40
living experiments 12

mandatory testing 11, 25-6, 105-9 133. *See also* screening
manipulation 74, 79
Mayo, David J. 108
McKusick, Leon 84, 88
McMearn, James 91-2
McNeil, Taylor 128
Medicaid 53
medical students 131-2
Mill, John Stuart 10, 12-13, 25, 135n22, 170n4
Mohr, Richard D. 20n25, 21n28, 36-7, 46, 56n6, 60n40, 97nn1,2, 138, 144-50, 155, 171n13
Mohr's argument 144-50, 155
monogamy 58n23, 59n34, 166-7
Montagnier, Luc 6
moral duty 11, 31-4, 44, 55, 57n13, 117
moral expectations 31-6, 40-4, 59n33. *See also* duty to disclose
moral imagination 13
moral responsibility 11, 30-6, 40-6, 137
moral worthiness 24, 103
multiple anonymous sex 37, 58n23, 59n33, 79, 122, 165-6. *See also* impersonal sex

Nadelmann, Ethan A. 123
narcotics 35, 82, 101, 118, 122-3, 140, 161-2, 170n6. *See also* IV drug-users
National Cancer Institute 6
need-based health care 151-4
needle-sharing 28-31, 90, 100n33, 118
New York 50, 164
"nothing can be done" argument 130
novus actus intervenens 57n10
nursing care 144-5, 147-51, 155.

options 11, 20n24, 64-5, 93, 103, 156, 167-8

Pasteur Institute 6
paternalistic legislation 56n3, 82-3, 122-4
PCP. *See* Pneumocystis carinii pneumonia
personal integrity 160
Pneumocystis carinii pneumonia 5, 7
positive discrimination 141. *See also* affirmative action
preferential health care 152-3
preferential hiring 141-2
Presidential Commission on the HIV Epidemic 112
Preston, John 59n32
prisons 37, 58nn24-26
privacy 66, 82, 105-6, 109, 111, 159
prohibition of narcotic use 91, 142, 170n5
psychoanalysis 173n32
psychological oppression 65, 79, 98nn9,10
psychotherapy 147, 163

public health 26, 46-52, 60n43, 106-7; economic and social costs of 53-5
public health authorities 90
public health ethic 48

quarantine 11, 105, 108, 109, 112

racism 18, 91-2, 124, 168, 170n6. *See also* discrimination
rape, homosexual 37-8, 46, 58n24
Rawls, John 124,
Rays family 112
Raz, Joseph 20n24,
Rechy, John 76-7
ribavirin 9
running partners 80-1

Sacramento, Calif. 85
safe sex (safer sex) 38, 39, 41-4, 52, 58n23, 59nn30,32, 67-8, 83, 85, 98n16, 163, 168
San Francisco 41, 50, 84-8, 100n41, 164
San Francisco Chronicle 85
San Francisco Health Department 84-5
Scotland 130-1
screening 7, 22, 106-9. *See also* mandatory testing
second-order desires 63
self-determination 66. *See also under* autonomy
self-esteem 16, 65, 92-3, 113, 119, 124-7, 132, 135nn26,28, 144, 147, 155-6, 160
self-inflicted harm. *See* harm to self
sexism 20n18
Shilts, Randy 19n9
shooting galleries 80-2, 140

social attitudes about gay men 75, 94, 131. *See also under* discrimination
social contamination 46, 49-51
social harms against gay men and IV drug-users 93-6, 117-20, 123-4, 133, 143-4, 168-9
social policy. *See* legislation and social policy
socially induced desires 105, 116-21
Somerville, Margaret 20n18
state-funded health care 16, 49, 139, 151-4
sterilized equipment 101n56
stigmatized groups 1-2, 17
strong harm principle 25, 56n3, 61, 104, 124, 137
Surgeon General's Report on AIDS 46

Third International Conference on AIDS 111
Titmuss, Richard M. 135n21
transmission of HIV/AIDS *See under* HIV/AIDS
trust 32-6, 57n14, 75, 87

United Kingdom 6
United States 6, 9, 28, 53, 84, 91, 111, 123, 142, 154-6, 159; Department of Justice 128; Supreme Court 129. *See also* Bowers v. Hardwick
University of Lethbridge, Canada 110
unsafe sex 41, 44, 52, 59n30, 99n21. *See also under* gay men
utilitarianism 170n4

volenti non fit injuria maxim 27, 30, 38, 45

voluntary action 36-7
voluntary associations 97n2

Ward, Elizabeth 152
weak harm principle 25, 56n3, 61-
 2, 66-7, 93, 104, 113-16, 124, 137
Weinberg, Martin S. 75, 94
Wilson, Harold 57n15
worried-well 2

Young, Robert 97n3
yuppie-desires 116-17, 119-20. *See
 also* BMW-desire

zidovudine. *See* azidothymidine